To Dr. Schroeder
Thanks for toturing
such good care me
Florence
Byrd

You're the Lord that Healeth...

You're the Lord that Healeth...

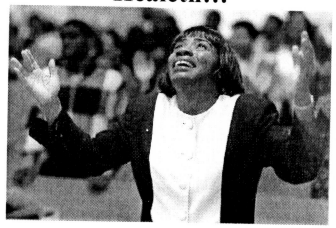

By
FLORENCE DYER

FLO'S PRODUCTIONS PUBLISHING SERVICE
An Affiliate of Writers & Self Publishers Association

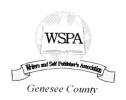

Genesee County

Unless otherwise indicated, all Old and New Testament Scriptures quotations are taken from the New King James Version of the Bible.

Scriptures quotations marked KJV are taken from the King James Version of the Bible.

First Published by AuthorHouse 11/24/04
Revised by Flo's Productions 11/15/05
Website: http://flosproductions.nstemp.biz
Email: florencedyer@comcast.net
(810) 334-2837

Manuscript and Project by Florence Dyer
Cover Design front & back Photographs
by Flint Journal Photographer Stuart Bauer
Quotations by Flint Journal Staff Writer Rose Mary Reiz
Front & Back Cover Designed by Flo's Productions

ISBN 0-9769645-3-8

Printed in the United States of America

FLORENCE DYER

I am the Lord that Healeth thee (Exodus 15:26 KJV)

You're the Lord that Healeth...

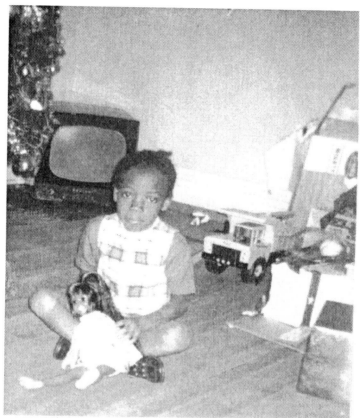

(Christmas 1969, Chicago, Ill Florence at age four)

I could not have imagined at such a young age, I'd undergo all the transitions, trials and tribulations that were awaiting me in my future. Sitting, daydreaming and playing with my dolls, could only be the ideal pleasure paradise, of a four year old. This photograph was taken a few months before my fifth birthday. Shortly after I turned five, the first transition in my life occurred, with my parent's permanent separation. -Florence Dyer

You're the Lord that Healeth...

Acknowledgements

I give all the honor, glory and praises to God; for He is the Creator of all Heaven and Earth. I would like to thank Him for creating both of my parents, my father Rev. Frank Phillips, Jr. and my mother the Late Verta Mae Phillips. Throughout my life the both of them have shown me unconditional love. Because of the two of them I have a strong faith and solid foundation in God. They've both shown me that I can be anything in life I want to be. I also thank the Lord for such a wonderful step-mother (Betsy) for her words of encouragement throughout the years. You have really been a blessing to me. Thank you for your advice, Godly wisdom, guidance and Godly direction.

I want to give a standing ovation to my loving husband Ted Alan Dyer for your unconditional love, commitment and support. I want to thank our two children Daniel and Patricia. Your beautiful little faces gave me the courage to succeed. You both have been through so much with me; you both are truly a blessing. I want to thank my eight siblings, Dorothy, Frank, Floyd, Frederick, Baton, Felexis, Lakeshia, and Benson. All of you have made my life very interesting. I love every one of you so much.

Friends and Family: Arthur and (Brenda) Parnell; Arthur is a fellow transplant recipient and a dear friend. Thanks to Elder John and Edra Thornton, you both have been such great friends through out the years. I value your friendship, your love and your support. Special thanks to the NJFGBC Nurses Guild, Health care Team (our President Marsha Hill and her husband Deacon George Hill). Special thanks to the Day Mission at NJFGBC. A special thanks to Sister Jollie Fields for your kindness, love and support. Thanks to Bishop Odis A. Floyd and the New Jerusalem Full Gospel Baptist Church Family. Special thanks to Norman and Michelle Gurley, Gina McMullen, Blanche, Michelle, Vanessa, Delores Holbrook, Beverly Polk, Maxine Hill, Phillip, Casandra and Brandi Miller, Gail Manning, Delores Johnson, Bessie R. Williams, Minister A. Jeffrey LaValley, Minister Gladys Scott, Minister Brenda Echols-Smith, Minister Ackor, Pastors Timothy and Tonya Stokes and Family Worship Church, Pastor Nathaniel and (Mother) Louis, the entire Gate Of Heaven Church Family, my cousin Bobbie J. Whitfield, Special friend Harryetta Mays, Minister Lynn Luelen, Sheila Clevenger, Glenn Morse, Douglas Whitehead, Elder Jennifer Scott, Evelyn Tyler, Ben Wilkerson, Mr. Quinton Garland, Billy

Simms, Danette Jenkins, Ken Milito, Matthew Lentz, Monique *(Mo)* Dewar-Ditari, Linda Trimble, Sharon Thomas, Kimberly and all the students at (UOP) University Of Phoenix, Cassandra Smith, brother-in-law and sister-in-law (Alfred and Gail Williams), Aunt Jackie, Aunt Mattie, (Cousins) Melinda, little "Dee Dee," Special friends Mac and Mary Davis.

Late Friends, Family & Pastor: Pastor Constance *("Pastor Connie")* Wilkerson. Your memory will last forever in my heart. Your spirit is so dearly missed. To one of my best friends and fellow Artist the late Demetrous McEwen, you were always rushing me out of the dialysis chair, you save a seat for me in glory I miss you my friend and brother in Christ. I want to thank the late Vera Augustine for her wonderful ham sandwiches she always made each treatments very interesting. My very special and dear friend the late Nanette, she inspired me to become a self-care patient. It is because of you I was able to take charge of my treatments. Your memory will live on in my heart always.

I would like to honor my late Aunt Evelyn Johnson, Uncle Roosevelt Hopkins, Uncle Milton Hopkins, Cousin Maxine Phillips, Cousins Diane, and Bruce your special memories will live on forever in my heart.

I would like to honor the Late ESRD Patients & family: my Grandfather Frank Phillips, Sr. Grandmother Florence Ella Hopkins, and my mothers oldest sister; Aunt Aileen Phillips.

I want to give a standing ovation to all of the dialysis staff and kidney transplant coordinators, health care professionals that made my transition run as smoothly as possible: (UOM) University Of Michigan Healthcare Systems (Ann Arbor, MI), Baxter (CAPD) Dialysis Supplies, Hurley Medical Center RDC Renal Dialysis Center, Hurley Park Plaza Dialysis Unit and McLaren Kidney Center.

I want to give a standing ovation to the entire Nephrologist staff of Doctors that have treated me over the past twenty years: Dr. Eliesha Singson, Dr. Paul Schroeder, Dr. Nabil Zaki, Dr. Sayed Osama, Dr. Odwa, Dr. Alumit, and Dr. Sergio Ponze. Dr. Ponze I want you to know that I have always respected your advice, even when we didn't always see eye-to-eye. You're an extraordinary doctor and a great friend. I know that you only care about my well-being.

Hurley Park Plaza Dialysis Nurses: Rutha Smith (You are a great friend and neighbor, thanks for believing in me God bless you), Cilia, (one of the first nurses that helped me make the transition to hemodialysis). Denise (thanks for tutoring me through my medical terminology class), Pam, Tracy, Falley Singson, Rene and Rita. Thanks to Hurley Medical Center social workers (Ladalia Postell, Susan Moon and Evelyn Clark). Thanks Tanesa Martin for being a blessing to my husband and me.

McLaren Kidney Center: I want to thank Angie and Sue for making my transition to the (CAPD) Continuous Ambulatory Peritoneal Dialysis training a smooth process. All of the nurses have not only been wonderful nurses in taking care of me; they've been great friends throughout the years. I love each one of you all so much. You all had a difficult job of putting up with me week after week but I could not have made it without you.

College Instructors: Dr. Philomenia *("Dr. Phil")* McPree Brown, *you have encouraged me to have the guts to write this book.* Dr. Joan Martin, you have encouraged me to have a love and a passion for *Literature.* Dr. Charles Totten thanks for introducing me to a world of great books. Michael Rucks, you gave me a clear understanding on human relations. Richard *("Rich")* Tesner, *you're one of the best Graphic Design Instructors.* It is because of you that I am the designer that I've become today. Thanks to the (UOP) University Of Phoenix, and the entire Baker College-Flint Staff.

Dez Martin, thank you for your words of encouragement throughout the years. You have always been a great friend and phlebotomius. Mrs. Semaj Brown thanks for your priceless advice and Godly wisdom. I thank the Lord for placing your kind giving spirit into my pathway. May He continue to richly bless you and Dr. Brown in all your future endeavors.

I have had the opportunity to work with some great people throughout the years. I would like to thank all my former employers: Catalyst Healthcare Group: Terri, Joe and Marge. Thanks for giving me an opportunity to work right out of medical school. Dr. Kimler, Electra Med Corporation, New Jerusalem FGBC, The McLaren Healthcare Corporation, Graphics Department: John Tracy, William, Ted, I want you all to know that you were great in showing me how to learn how to use the computer without the mouse. John you would be very proud to see that I don't use the mouse all the time. Thanks to Ted for showing me how to take pictures with a digital camera. I have taken Williams advice about sketching continuously. Although I love graphics it will never replace a hand drawn sketch. I still find myself sketching all the time. I want to also take the opportunity to thank the late Dr. Heller. Who had always shown me so much kindness.

There are so many people to thank and it is so hard to acknowledge everyone by name. However, if I've forgotten to mention your name it was not done so on purpose. I would like to take this time to extend my gratitude for all that you've done, I love you all and thank God I have had the opportunity to connect with you in some way.

I believe what (Prov. 17:17) says about a friend: *A friend loveth at all times, and a brother is born for adversity.*

There are so many people that have deposited so much into my life. It is because of the kindness shown by each one of you I have been shaped and molded into the person I have become today. During numerous adversities in my life the support and kindness of friendly gestures have exceeded my expectations (Job 6:14 Amplified) gives an excellent example of the kindness of friends shown during his greatest calamity:

To him who is about to faint and despair, kindness is due from his friends, lest he forsake the fear of the Almighty.

I would like to extend a special thanks to Dr. Stevens for the earlier medical care he provided to my brother and me. Special thanks to the Fresenius Medical Care Nurses for administering the Plasmapheresis treatments: Thanks Melody, Pam, Leigh Diamond and David Marcozzi for all the very interesting conversations. The four of you helped to keep my mind at ease during each of the Plasmapheresis treatments. God Bless you all. You are very special people.

A Special thanks to Officer David Dicks for sitting in while I underwent the Plasmapheresis treatments. Thanks for doing such a great job hosting the WSPA Book Review Show.

Thanks to the Gift of Life and The Hurley Foundation for purchasing my Rapamune Anti Rejection Medication. I would like to thank the Rapamune Patient Assistant Program for assisting me with getting my medicine. The Patient Assist representative Scott took the time to address all of my concerns. A Special thanks goes to Karen from the ChampVA Meds-By-Mail Pharmacy (for rushing the Rapamune Anti Rejection medication right away). You are angels sent from heaven.

I want to also thank all the Journalist for their help in raising awareness about the lifestyle struggles of ESRD patients. Special thanks to Flint Journal Staff Writers Rose Mary Reiz, George Jaksa and Common Ground talk show host Walethia Coleman.

FLORENCE DYER

Dedication

To the Lord of my life *Jehovah Rophi* my Healer, you're my *El Shaddai* a God of more than enough for me.

To all the ESRD patients I've being acquainted with throughout the years and ESRD patients around the world.

To the three most important people in my life; my husband Ted and our two children Daniel and Patricia. Everyday with you three gives me a reason to get up and keep going on each day.

Table Of Contents

FLORENCE DYER

Prologue

*You're the Lord that Healeth...*is a book that has been long overdue. For years various friends suggested, I write about my experiences. But it took some time for me to really consider the idea. When I finally gave the idea some thought, it became a great challenge for me in knowing where and how to begin. Whenever there is a project I'm considering, I always want to give myself to it completely. Any design I create becomes a true extension of myself. Writing this book is no different than the process I use, for producing my designs.

My ultimate purpose was to produce a product that would be a true reflection of my experiences with enduring *Hemodialysis, Peritoneal Dialysis,* receiving a *Cadaver Kidney Transplant* and receiving a *Related Kidney Transplant.* Over the past twenty years I have been through so much, it was difficult to know where to begin. There were numerous times I attempted to sit down and write about my experiences but it was too painful to look back. It was really hard to think about a lot of the losses. Most importantly I did not want to leave any stone unturned that would be helpful to other (ESRD) End Stage Renal Disease patients.

Well finally I decided, if I was going to write about my experiences it was best to let go and let God. That is the way I have always lived my life and was not about to stop now. The most frustrating thing I discovered was opening a lot of old wounds. There was so much locked up on the inside of me, once I started writing all of it began pouring out at once. After letting the information flow naturally, organizing it all seemed to be another great challenge.

*You're the Lord that Healeth...*covers a lot of issues. Throughout the eighteen chapters I express how I dealt with enduring each form of treatment. Going through dialysis for the first time can be a very eye opening experience. After the first few treatments patients generally get familiar with the regular routine. While on the other hand waiting on a cadaver kidney organ can be

1

very frustrating. You simply don't know if it will happen for you. You also don't know how things will turn out if it does happen. This frustration can be alleviated depending upon how a patient spends their wait. The more the wait on a cadaver organ is the focal point in a patient's life, the more frustrated the patient will become. But if the patient allows things to happen, as they will in God's own time, they'll make the transition go a lot more smoothly.

"Educate While You Wait"

While undergoing hemodialysis it was important for me to educate myself the entire time. I felt if I was going to be undergoing the treatments it was best to learn everything about dialysis. Even though I learned a lot of things, it did not seem like the things I'd learned would one day benefit anyone else. I thought of going through hemodialysis as just something I had to do in order to survive. I never would have thought my experiences would one-day amount to anything worth writing or reading about. But now looking back at all that I have lived through, I've began to realize how blessed I truly am.

After enduring years of hemodialysis, (CAPD) Continuous Ambulatory Peritoneal Dialysis and surviving two kidney transplant operations; I think each of these experiences qualifies me to speak about each form of treatment. It is amazing how we go through very trying ordeals in our lives and come out still standing? I am one to never believe God causes theses adversities, but He will bring us out of them.

In fact (Psm. 46:11) says, *God is our refuge and strength a very present help in trouble.* All we have to do is call on Him, which lead me to (Jeremiah 33:3) where God said, *call unto Me, and I will answer thee and shew thee great and mighty things, which thou knowest not.*

Forward

*You're The Lord that Healeth...*was birthed out of a lot of hurt, pain, and devastation. First of all, I have battled with (ESRD) End Stage Renal Disease for over twenty years. Secondly, I've lost a lot of close friends to ESRD. Finally, both of my grandparents died from ESRD. My grandmother died six years, before I was born. During the late 50's, my grandmother (Florence Ella Hopkins) was diagnosed with ESRD. During her time, doctors were not fully aware of how to treat ESRD. Over 40 years ago, dialysis treatments were still fairly new to the medical profession. The new experimental treatments were also extremely expensive. Because of the costly treatments, dialysis was only being offered to a select few (*Patients that could afford the treatments).* Being a woman of modest means, my grandmother was not among the select few.

I've spoke with several patients who had undergone treatments, during the late 50's. They're very impressed, with all the advancements in dialysis and kidney transplants. One (TRFH) transplant recipient/former hemodialysis patient told me, *"in the beginning trials of hemodialysis, patients had to undergo 24-hour treatments. Because of the lengthy treatments, patients had to be hospitalized."*

Another (TRFH) patient said, *"he had to stay overnight several days a week."* Even a former CAPD patient shared, *"how uncomfortable the catheter tubing was for him. Gradually each treatment advanced to the place, where patients were given better options. The improvements in administering treatments, allowed patients the option of choosing to dialysis at home or in a dialysis unit."*

Wow, I love America! We live in the greatest country in the world. It is a blessing to live in such a time as now. Where the research in the progression of dialysis treatments, and kidney transplants has come a long ways. Scientist are making improvements in technology all the time. Dialysis patients are living a lot longer and feeling a lot better. In fact, most are living more productive lifestyles. Doctors have better methods on how to treat organ transplant rejection. The anti-rejection medications are monitored a lot more closely. The organ transplant operations are much more sophisticated. The *Recipients* and *Donors* are treated with the best surgical techniques available on the market today. If it was any time to receive a kidney transplanted organ the time is now.

Even though technology has advanced, there is one thing about Cadaver Kidney Organ donations that have remained constant. There is still a massive shortage of *"Donors."* There are more patients in need of transplanted organs, than there are donors willing to donate organs. The waiting list for a cadaver kidney organ can be anywhere from 3-7 years. There are a lot of patients who die while waiting.

ESRD has no special race, in which it has chosen to strike. However, there are far more African American patients on dialysis than any other race. In addition, to the increase of African American ESRD patients on dialysis, there's a lack of African Americans getting involved in a solution. African Americans are really the most notorious race about not donating organs. These are devastating facts to talk about; especially since I am an African American. But I have to put the facts out there anyways. In spite, of the massive donor shortage, scientists are still working relentlessly for other options.

There has been another new breakthrough in the area of organ transplants. Scientist are making it possible for patients to receive Living Donor Kidney Transplants from donors with blood types different from their own. According to a recent study conducted by the Rochester Mayo Clinic, there are about 45,000 patients waiting for a Cadaver Kidney Organ in the United States. About 8,000 kidneys are available each year. However, about 7,000 patients who are waiting for an organ are infected with elevated antibodies. **Elevated antibodies:** *is a rise in proteins produced by the body, which reacts specifically with a foreign substance in the body.*

In the pass five years doctors have started treating elevated antibodies with Plasmapheresis treatments. I will mention more about Plasmapheresis in chapter 18.

Patients with elevated antibodies make a kidney-transplanted organ more likely to fail. There are two new types of organ transplant procedures that's making kidney transplants an option for thousands in waiting. The progression has occurred in the area of ABO-Incompatible Living Donor Transplants and the Positive Crossmatch Transplants. Both areas has made science move one step closer to another discovery of "Xenotransplantation" (pig to human transplant) a reality. – According to Dr. Stegall (Mayo Clinic Researchers for kidney and pancreas transplants).

I have presented the results from the Mayo Clinics research. The research covers the options available through the area of *ABO-Incompatible Living Donor Transplants* and *Positive Crossmatch Transplants* and *Xenotransplantation*. I am in no way trying to endorse a patient's decision in making a choice for considering a *Positive Crossmatch, ABO-Incompatible Living Donor Transplants* organ or *Xenotransplantation*. However, it is better for patients to be informed about all new options that are available. There are so many patients dying, because of the massive donation shortage. Therefore, I commend scientist for all their efforts. I am always mindful of how far we've come.

I attended a kidney transplant conference several years ago. During the conference doctors announced *"Xenotransplantation"* as another one of the latest research studies for kidney transplants. At that time the thought of receiving a *"Pig's Organ"* was too frightening for me to even think about. I'm still not too keen on the idea for myself. This is my own personal preference. However, the possibility of the procedure happening is not too far off from becoming a reality for other patients. Over the past forty years, there has been so much progression in each form of treatment. Therefore, it is difficult for anyone to be very adamant about sticking with one form of treatment. We are very fickle minded beings and can never say, what we will or will not do.

I can remember saying to myself, there is no way I'll ever have a kidney transplant. Well not only did I have one kidney transplant; now I've had two. I was on hemodialysis a little over three years before I made up my mind, to get on the cadaver transplant list. Fortunately, my wait on the cadaver kidney was nine months. When the cadaver kidney came available, I did not have elevated antibodies. Not all patients have been as fortunate.

"Choosing The Best Treatment Option"

As with any form of treatment you choose, you'll need to weigh the pros and cons of each one. Afterwards, select the treatment that is best for you. There are three forms of treatments available for ESRD patients.

The three forms of treatment available are:

Form Of Treatment	Methods
Hemodialysis	(Dialysis in a nearby unit or Home Hemodialysis
Two Types of *Peritoneal Dialysis*	(CAPD) Continuous Ambulatory Peritoneal Dialysis or (CCPD) Continuous Cycling Peritoneal Dialysis
The *kidney* **Transplant**	(Cadaver Kidney Transplant, Related Transplant and a live unrelated kidney transplant).

I have been fortunate to have endured all three methods available. One thing which cannot be overlooked, I'm still alive to discuss each one of them. Not every patient has the same experience, with either form of treatment. There are good and bad experiences with each form of treatment. Therefore, another patients experience does not have to be your experience.

Even though my brother and I were diagnosised with the same kidney disease "Glomeronephritis" we have not been affected in the same way. I have experienced some symptoms that he hasn't. He has also experienced symptoms that I haven't. Therefore, you cannot judge your experience by someone else's, even if they are related to you. Every person is unique in there own way. There are certain anti-rejection medications that I can't take. However, these same medications work just fine for other kidney transplant patients. That is why it is important to gather as much information from other patients. Although, you gather the information analyze it. Don't automatically think you'll experience the same reaction in your case. Pray about the situation first. Always make your choices, based on the treatment that is best for you.

I am not writing this book to tell you what to do. I am writing to give you my experience. Hopefully, you'll determine from what I have lived through, that you'll endure too. Your life does not have to end because you've been diagnosised with ESRD. *Your life is what you make it.* It is my deepest hope that patients walk away from reading this book, with the greatest of expectations for conquering everything in their lives. Patients can live productive, fully enriched lifestyles, even though they have ESRD. Always remember, there are ESRD patients living productive lives everyday. It is not just my brother and I.

I also felt compelled to write this book because there are so many hurting people in the world. When you're going through something for the first time, it can be very frightening. It is always more comforting, to find someone that can relate to what you're going through. Although, our families live with us, they don't truly know us. While on the other hand, it is important to know that ESRD affects everyone around you. There are adjustments that have to be made, to accommodate any form of treatment. It doesn't matter if you're undergoing dialysis or if you've had a kidney transplant. The emotional adjustment can be a very slow process. Even though our families can be emotionally supportive they cannot take the pain and frustration away. This is something only the Lord can do.

It always helps to have someone that you can talk too, in the down times. Most of the time, you'll just have to cry out to the Lord. There will be times they're no words to express how you feel. However, there are other techniques that can help you deal with what you're experiencing. Start keeping a journal and writing down how you feel each day. You'll be surprised down the road at the amazing changes that will have taken place. When you began to reflect back over your experience, you'll no longer be the same person anymore.

When I started putting together *You're the Lord that Healeth...* I came across a lot of old notes, essays and journals I had written throughout the years. It was really fascinating to see how I had grown, throughout each stage in my life. What I was going through at one stage encouraged me when it was time to go through a similar incident. A lot of times how you handle one event can help you through a similar situation in your future. Just writing this book alone has been so therapeutic for me. I've heard people say how writing a book released a lot of their pain. I know that writing has helped me to release years of pent-up frustrations.

Therefore, if you have been diagnosised with ESRD and have to receive any form of treatment, you'll find the information contained in *You're the Lord that Healeth...* very informative.

I am sure from time to time you might even have to refer back to it, throughout your waiting process. Whatever the case, I hope that *You're the Lord that Healeth...* will be a blessing to you. Most importantly it is my prayer that you don't limit God's way of blessing you. Your healing may include the use of medicine or professional intervention. Continue to pray and trust in the Lord for your healing. When you receive an answer from the Lord you will know it. No doctor in the world will have to tell you anything. Keep in mind (Rom.8:28) *And we know all things work together for the good to them that love God, to them who are called according to His purpose.*

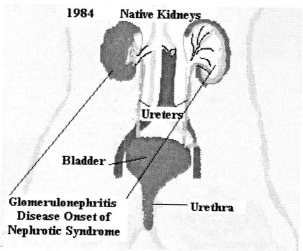

1984 Native Kidneys

Ureters

Bladder

Glomerulonephritis
Disease Onset of
Nephrotic Syndrome

Urethra

Photograph drawn by Florence Dyer

1

Hearing The Diagnosis

Yea, though I walk through the valley of the shadow of death, I will fear no evil; for thou art with me; thy rod and thy staff they comfort me (Psm. 23:4).

The summer of 1984

Is the year my life completely changed forever. I awoke early, feeling very disoriented one extremely hot summer day. I sat on the side of the bed until eventually containing my composure. Even with the unusual symptoms, I was completely obvious to the next few moments being the most horrifying experience of my life. This day will forever edged into my memory.

Eventually, I staggered into the bathroom to wash my face. I began to run the cold water as I reached for a face towel. Barely awake, I glanced into the mirror. At the first glimpse, it was as if I was looking at a disfigure creature. I was still feeling a little drowsy and barely awake. I continued to run the water over the face towel repetitively ringing the towel out. After I covered my face with the dampened face rag, I slowly removed the towel to sneak a peek into the mirror once again. Bracing my cheeks in the palm of my hands, I began to scream at the face I saw. It was as if I was living in a nightmare. This led me to wonder if I was really awake. There were enormous bags hanging down from what once were my normal eyelids. As I tried to brace myself I immediately glanced down at my feet. Both of my ankles and feet were like inflated balloons. They were so swollen, I could hardly maintain my balance.

Totally distraught, I hobbled over to the phone as fast as I could. It was at that very moment my family doctors (Doctor Stevens) phone number seemed to be readily apparent in my mind. I was never one that liked to go to the doctor. But I had no problem in going now. After the receptionist picked up the phone, I immediately began to spout off nervously telling her about the horrible site I saw in the mirror. She was barely able to get a word in edge wise. I'm certain she could hear the desperation in my voice. Finally, after taking a breath she was able to speak. She said, *"I'll look at Dr. Stevens schedule and possibly squeeze you in."* *"However even if she squeezed me in, it would be a long wait because he was booked solid for the day."* Before I could respond, *"She said hold please."* and she placed me on hold.

While waiting to confirm the appointment my heart started racing so fast. At this point, I was completely petrified in the midst of waiting for her to return. I was holding the phone in one hand and trying to get dressed at the same time. This was very terrifying for me because I had never had so much as a common cold. Doctors were not exactly my cup of tea either. There was not a clue in my mind as to what was going on.

"Making The Connection"

I had a younger brother that had been diagnosised with a kidney disease earlier in the same year. This never dawned on me, I could be experiencing the same thing. All I knew was that I wanted the swelling to go down as soon as possible. Other than that I was not able to put too many other concrete thoughts together. I was frustrated from trying to buckle up my sandals. The receptionist returned to the phone and said *"Dr. Stevens would see me but I would have to wait for a while to be seen."* *"I told her fine as long as it was today."* I was happy just to get into the doctors office. I don't even remember saying good bye.

After quickly hanging up the phone, the only thoughts running through my mind were the concerns about how could this happen to me? What did I do? And finally if I was going to die? I was trying to think about what I ate that could have caused this. After trying on several other pairs of sandals, eventually I said the heck with it. I decided to slip on a pair of footees. All I knew is that, I needed to get to the doctor as soon as possible. It seemed like I could not get out of the house fast enough. With all the commotion it is amazing no one in the house woke up. I left so fast I did not wake up my mother or say anything to anybody.

Once I arrived at the doctor's office, I checked in and sat down. Dr. Stevens was very familiar with my family history. Once inside of the examining room Doctor Stevens without any hesitation said, *"my symptoms reminded him of my brother Floyd's symptoms."*

I was simply speechless by his response. Doctor Stevens had treated my Floyd and diagnosised him with having *Glomeronephritis.* Dr. Stevens said, in order for him to be 100% certain he was going to schedule a biopsy of my kidneys. It suddenly hit me, *my God the swelling should have really triggered a comparison to my brother's condition.* Even though the symptoms were similar, I did not want to even consider having any condition. My mind began to wonder if I had made the right choice, in coming to the same doctor. This was the same doctor that treated my brother with steroids. The steroids made my brother blow up and look even more disfigured. Well for the moment, I was experiencing a lot of the disfigurement without the steroids. Therefore I remained calm about my choice.

Doctor Stevens said, *"there was not much he could do for me at this time."* *"Until the other test were completed he would prescribe water pills to drain the fluid off of my feet and ankles."*

He said, *"the water pills would also make the swelling in my eyelids go down too."* This made me feel a little more comfortable. At least I would be able to wear my shoes again. In addition, to my face not looking so horrific either. I left Doctor Stevens office totally in shock. He told me none of the things I wanted to hear.

I immediately got the prescription filled at the nearest pharmacy. While waiting for the prescription to get filled, thoughts were racing through my mind. I was still thinking, maybe I ate the wrong food. Maybe after I take the medicine everything would disappear and soon I'd return back to normal. Once arriving back home I immediately told my mom what Doctor Stevens said. She was completely petrified at hearing the news and she was horrified with how I looked too. She had really just come to grips with my bothers condition and she seemed to be totally speechless. Just the thought of one of her children being stricken with a dreadful disease was too much. Now she had to probably face another one of her children undergoing the same prognosis. After telling my mom, I eventually called my dad in Chicago. He offered to take me to a specialist in Chicago to have the biopsy done. My dad did not hesitate to drive up and get me as soon as possible.

My dad scheduled and appointment with a specialist close to his home. The specialist ordered lab work and the biopsy. After I had the biopsy procedure done, the specialist said *"I would receive the results in a few days."* All I could think about was having several more days, I did not know what was going on. I did not even want to consider the prognosis Dr. Stevens gave me. After the biopsy results came back, the specialist confirmed I had Glomeronephritis (a rare incurable kidney disease). What I felt most was total shock and dismay; my mind was so perplexed, I did not know how to react to the news. Therefore, I did not react verbally at all. It was as if, at that very moment my body went completely numb. The specialist continued to let me know; there was a disintegration of the disease called *"Nephritic Syndrome"* which had already begun the process of eating away at my kidney function.

The Doctor broke down the terminology to explain how a process called *nephritic syndrome* was eating up my kidney function. He said, *"the process is completely irreversible and over time, my kidney function would totally dissolve."* The doctor estimated the entire process, would probably take about fifteen years (before the deterioration was complete). He said, *"it was without a doubt I would definitely have to undergo dialysis treatments or I will die."* Hearing him say those words was as if at that very moment, I had died right then. He continued on to say, *"either I would have to undergo dialysis treatments or receive a kidney transplant, in order to remain alive."* From that point on, I can't really remember if my dad asked more questions or if I did. I can only recall how I felt which was totally Helpless.

How does a nineteen year old handle a doctor saying, *"you have an incurable disease?"* To me it is totally inconceivable to even imagine. (*You have an incurable disease*) is not five words anyone wants to hear out of the mouth of a doctor. To top it all off, no one wants to even think about *dying.* He cleared up any misconception I could possibly have. When he said, *the kidney would continue to shrink until all of the function completely deteriorated. The most frightening part of it all there was nothing that could be done about it.* Asking the question of how it started was totally beyond their understanding. The doctors did not know how it started or where it came from. The only certainty he had was it is definitely irreversible. This did not leave me much hope.

It was devastating for me, to one-day wake up and have my life completely turned upside down. Before the diagnosis, I was a totally healthy person. There was not even a cause or reason doctors could give me for this long foreign word *Glomeronephritis.* A word I could barely pronounce.

The specialist wanted to start treating me with large dosages of *Prednisone.* This was not appealing to me at all. These were the same steroids prescribed to treat my brother. *I told the doctor no thanks; I saw what happened to my brother.* My brother's kidney function completely deteriorated the moment he

13

began taking steroids. In fact, Floyd was at the point of getting ready to start hemodialysis treatments any day.

Even though I refused the steroids, I was willing to do whatever else; I could to maintain the function I had left. I asked the doctor, *"if he had something else he could recommend."* He told me, *"as long as I stayed away from salt, monitored my blood pressure and managed my weight, I could sustain my function for a long time. However, even if I followed all the preventive measures to the letter, I must face the inevitable. Dialysis was going to be unavoidable."* He went on to say, *"no matter what I did or how good I managed my salt intake, or watched out for all the other areas one day in the future I would be starting dialysis. He recommended I follow-up with a Nephrologist upon returning back to Flint."*

Once I left the hospital, I did not even want to think about what the doctor told me. I was young and by that time the swelling in my feet and ankles were back down. I left the hospital thinking, that doctor did not know what he was talking about. I decided to live with my dad for a while. I returned back to Flint about six months later. Even though I was in denial I managed to follow most of what the doctor prescribed. Although, I did not want to adhere to all of the doctor's advice, I did stop eating salt, monitored my blood pressure and maintained my weight. Eventually when I got home, I followed up with a Nephrologist.

Upon my return, later in the same year I began dating a former boyfriend. We met shortly after I graduated high school. It was important for me to resume as much of a normal life as possible. For once I began thinking about my future. I even considered the possibility of marriage and children. The Nephrologist (in Flint) told me I would probably never be able to have children. Shows how wrong the doctor was. In 1985 I became pregnant with my first child. The entire time I was pregnant with my son, I was at a high risk of going on dialysis. It was not surprising to me; since that was something I'd been told before. I followed up very closely with an Obstetrician (Dr. Burns). After the birth of my son, the Nephrologist told me, *"it would be best not to have any more children."* Eighteen months later, I gave birth to my daughter.

In 1987 I was twenty-three years old. It had been three years since, I was diagnosised with kidney disease. At the time of the diagnosis, I did not realize all the condition entailed. Looking back now, if I had listened to what the doctors told me, I would have missed out on the two greatest joys in my life. *My two children are a real blessing.* (Psm. 127:3) says, *children are a heritage from the Lord; and the fruit of the womb is His reward.* It was for the both of them to be here. They are miracles. Although I had so many complications with the pregnancy of my daughter. In spite of it all I pulled through.

Immediately after giving birth to my daughter, I began to experience a lot of symptoms. I was having spinal headaches, and uncontrollable high blood pressure. During my stay in the hospital, the Obstetrician recommended my family doctor (Dr. Stevens) and a Nephrologist (Dr. Alumit) follow me up. Both doctors had great concerns about my systolic pressure remaining over 200 and my diastolic was over 100. Doctor Stevens said, *"the elevated BP was putting me at high risk of threatening a stroke. He recommended I remain hospitalized until the blood pressure became regulated."* Once my blood pressure stabilized, I was released from the hospital. I returned home for about one week. Until one night while feeding my daughter, I fell out unconscious. It was a blessing her dad was there to catch her. I was rushed back to the hospital in an ambulance. I woke up in the ICU Intensive Care Unit. The doctors asked, *"what did I remember before I passed out?"* I could barely remember anything. My last memory was about feeding my daughter. The doctors told me, *"I had experienced a seizure at home. Also I had experienced two more seizures when I arrived at the hospital."* I had no recollection of either one of the seizures.

During my stay in the hospital, the doctors once again were having problems stabilizing my blood pressure. However, now they were trying to figure out why I was also experiencing seizure disorder. The elevated blood pressure and seizure activity persisted off and on for about a month. I remain hospitalized, until doctors could come up with more concrete answers. Through the use of diuretics my blood pressure finally stabilized. The doctors were also treating the seizures with a drug called *Dilantin.* Once everything was controlled, the doctors discharged me from the hospital. Until this very day the doctors have never come up with a reason for the seizure disorder.

"Taking Charge Of My Life"

When I returned home, my children's dad and I began arguing all the time. It was one argument after another. Our main fight was over how the children should be raised. It was difficult enough coming home and getting acquainted with a new baby. Also I was caring for a very active eighteen month old. Their dad felt with my failing kidneys, the seizure disorders and problems with my blood pressure it would be best for his mother to raise our daughter. This was definitely out of the question. I did not want to think of either one of our children turning out like him. Their dad began drinking all the time. It was difficult enough dealing with him when he wasn't drinking. It was a living nightmare when he was. I have never been a drinker and this was way too much for me to handle. My children's father and I could not make it. Their dad's abuse of alcohol began to take a toll on our relationship. We broke up almost a year after I became better.

At first it was a struggle, when I began raising our children alone. However, this was one of the best decisions I ever made. Bringing up children in an abusive environment was not something, I wanted for them or myself. Most of all, the alcohol was not something I wanted around the children either. Their dad and I were arguing constantly even after we broke up. It was not an amicable parting. But I had reached a point in my life, that only making choices that were better for my health came first. There was no way I could tolerate a toxic relationship. I was not going to allow anything to speed up the deterioration of my remaining kidney function. I am glad we were never married, it would have made parting a lot worse. Although, we had plans of getting married I believe we made the right decision not to. When their dad and I were together he intentionally tried to do everything to sabotage my dreams. There was no way; I was going to allow anything or anyone to hold me down. This was my life and I was going to live it to the fullest. No way I was going to allow a person or disease any power of holding me from what the Lord was showing me. This was a power; I refused to give to another.

I did not allow ESRD to hold me back. I'll be darn if I was going to allow their dad to think he could. Out of their dad's bitterness about our breakup; he told me "*I would not live long anyways.*" These bitter parting words, only helped me to realize he was not the one for me. Often times I think about when I tried to attend college he'd promise to keep the children. He would wait right until it was time for me to register for classes, just so he could change his mind. For a couple years after I left their dad my health remained stable. I was so happy to be free of the toxic relationship. It was really hard to imagine I had stayed in the relationship so long. We were together for seven years. Although, I wasn't living right, I've always had a strong belief in God. With leaving him, I could now renew my relationship with the Lord.

"Never Get Too Relaxed In Doing Well"

In the mid part of 1990, I was twenty-five years old. My son was three and my daughter was almost two. I got accepted into the Medical Nursing Program (at the University Of Michigan Flint). I was so excited about my acceptance into the Medical Program. I arranged my schedule to attend classes a few days a week. I placed both of my children in a nearby day care. I was really excited about how things were going in my life. I never experienced any more seizures and my blood pressure was under control. For a long time, I had felt great.

Until one day, I got up to go to school and I passed out in my cousin Tim's apartment. My cousin immediately called the ambulance. I was rushed over to Hurley Medical Center. When I arrived at the emergency room, I began to gradually come around. Once I was completely awake the doctor came into the room. The emergency doctor said *"they had run a lot of test."* He went on to say, *"I needed to begin dialysis."* I told him *"Okay; I know about that already"* (I had a sort of smirk look on my face, like he wasn't telling me something I had not heard before). I went on to say, *"the Doctors have been telling me that for years. They told me I had Glomeronephritis."*

The doctor looked at me again to make sure I clearly understood what he was saying. (With a smart-alecky expression) I said, *"okay the doctors had already told me that before, so what else is new?"* (He could tell I didn't want to hear anything else he had to say. But he was anxious to grab my attention anyways).

He said, *"Miss I don't think you clearly understand what I am saying to you."* *"You need to begin dialysis right now! Or you're going to die."* He repeated himself with a little more inferences by saying, *"if you don't began dialysis treatments very soon you will die."* (He was looking directly into my eyes without any hesitation). It was at that very moment; it all began to settle in. I thought about this could be the end of the road for me.

The doctor said, *"he would schedule an appointment with a local Nephrologist, for me to receive a method for administering treatments as soon as possible."*

He discussed how the *"nephritis had eaten up most of my kidney function. At the present time, I had only about 10% of my kidney function left."* He continued on saying, *"my kidneys were no longer able to cleanse my blood enough to sustain my life. The poison had built up so high in my blood stream. This is why I passed out."* I sat there silently and I truly believe, this was the first time the reality of the kidney disease began to sink in. I knew if I did not take this seriously, I was going to die. Hearing another doctor say this for a third time is even more frightening then the first time. In fact, the third time was much worst than the other two. Before I was given a little more time. I had managed for seven years without treatments. It didn't matter how good I had managed, I never wanted to hear these words again.

It didn't matter what the doctors said, all I knew was that I did not want to die. I was just beginning to live my life. There was so much I had not done or seen. I was not happy about starting treatments, but I did not have much of a choice. It seemed from the time I received the report my symptoms began to get worse. In fact, it seemed like my health began to gradually deteriorate more and more each day. The worst I began to feel, the more it became apparent to me it was time to begin treatments.

Upon the deterioration of my kidney function, I began to categorically experience the following symptoms:

- Uncontrolled High Blood Pressure
- Memory loss
- Confusion (Unable to concentrate)
- Insomnia
- Depression
- Hair loss
- Weight loss
- Fatigue
- Muscle Weakness
- Breathing Apnea
- Dizziness
- Severe Anemia
- Swelling in my ankles, feet, and eyelids
- Itchy Dry skin
- Loss of Appetite
- Diarrhea
- Vomiting
- Decrease in Urine output

A lot of these symptoms may vary for each patient. Some of the symptoms might even be worst in one case and less severe in another. There are some ESRD patients whose symptoms might even be the complete opposite. For instance, when my kidneys failed I loss a lot of weight. While on the other hand, there were other patients that gained a lot of weight. Patients are different in how their body reacts to the effects of the disease. My kidneys could no longer remove any extra fluid intake, causing the extra fluid to collect into the tissues in my body. Although, my kidneys were failing, I was still producing urine output. Throughout the entire time of undergoing treatments, I continued to have urine output. *This is where most ESRD patients miss it.* They feel that since their bodies are still producing urine output, then they are okay. But soon they discover that even though the kidneys might still produce urine output, it does not mean the kidneys are healthy.

If a Pre-ESRD patient examines their urine output more closely, they would discover the urine is not like normal urine. The urine output does not even contain the same amount of waste products that it should. *"Denial can be a very stubborn enemy to Pre-ESRD patients."* The patient will begin at some point to realize the amount of urine output produced does not necessarily determine how well the kidneys are working. *"Quantity does not equal Quality."*

There are patients who might be experiencing all the symptoms I mentioned, but still choose to be in denial. I've been there before too. My earlier experience clearly demonstrates that. Even though you're experiencing the symptoms, it is your choice to still continue ignoring them. In spite, of all the information you've received there is one question; which may still loom your mind.

Why do I need dialysis?

The reason that you need dialysis is because when your kidneys were once healthy they worked 24 hours a day, 7 days a week to keep your body in balance. Whenever you ate or drunk, a lot of the important nutrients went into the bloodstream to be used as fuel to keep your body healthy. Your system functioned normally to keep the things that it needed to make you stay strong and healthy and it

20

would get rid of the things the body did not need. Now that your kidneys are no longer healthy the things that your body no longer needs are remaining in your bloodstream causing the body not to function properly. Dialysis is a way to clean your blood to help your body function the way it should.

After being discharged from HMC my symptoms began to get even worse. Everything from this point on seemed to go really fast. I kept my scheduled appointment with Dr. Alumit (a local Nephrologist). The Nephrologist referred me to a vascular surgeon. The vascular surgeon scheduled an emergency surgery, to install a small *arteriovenous fistula.* An arteriovenous fistula *is a surgical connection of an artery placed directly into a vein for the purpose of administering hemodialysis treatments.*

After having the surgical procedure there is a six-week waiting period for the fistula site to completely heal. During the waiting period, I began to get a lot weaker as the poison in my bloodstream began to rise. I experienced a huge loss of appetite and difficulty breathing. Everything I ate came back up and my hair started falling out. I lost over forty pounds in less than a month. I began to discover I could not make it without some form of divine intervention.

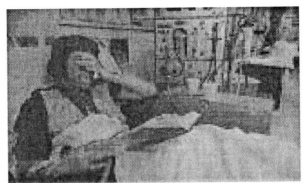

Photograph taken by Flint Journal Photographer Stuart Bauer

2

Starting Dialysis

Is anything too hard for the Lord? At the time appointed I will return until thee (Gen.18:14 a)

On June 29, 1991

I began hemodialysis treatments. At the time I was only twenty-six years old, barely a hundred pounds and a single mom. With my weight being so low, the Doctors ordered each treatment run for two hours and fifteen minutes. The quantity of a dialysis run depends on a patient's weight, and the amount of time it takes for a complete clearance of the toxins to be removed from the bloodstream. The dialysis nurses usually start patients out with the small artificial kidney as just a trial run. Then they generally would switch the patients to the larger kidney (maybe after a few runs). I used the small artificial kidney for a lot longer then usual because I did not weigh very much.

When I first began treatments, I did not want to see anyone or talk to anyone. A lot of the people at the dialysis unit were a lot older than me and it seemed as though we did not have a lot in common. Little did I know; we had way more than I could ever imagine. I could not help thinking about my children. My son had just turned four and my daughter was three in a half. Both of my children were still babies. My mom was keeping them on days I was undergoing treatments. I had to drop all of my classes at the University because I did not have the energy to keep up. All I kept thinking about was there is no way; I was going to spend my life this way. I would go into the bathroom before I began each treatment to pray for deliverance. I can remember a lot of prayers promising if I was delivered off of dialysis, how I would serve the Lord with all my heart. I can remember one of the prayers, where the Lord gave me an answer in my spirit saying, *"Start Right Now."* I was thinking once He healed my body than I would serve Him.

As I began to grow spiritually, and read my bible daily I discovered the Lord wants us to serve Him when we're going through; not just when things are going good. Through the word I began to trust Him even in the hard times. A lot of times when He instantly heals our bodies, we will slip back into our old ways. After coming into the understanding of the Lords Will for my life, I began to tell of His goodness while I was at the dialysis unit. Soon I began to tell of His goodness everywhere I went. After a while the Lord led me to a church home. Once I fully committed life to the Lord, I started to see my faith was growing stronger. There is no way a person can be touched by the Lord and remain the same, it is impossible. My relationship with the Lord made me better able to deal with what I was experiencing. Soon dialysis became a temporary thing I had to do. I truly believed one day I'd be delivered, so even now I was going to enjoy life. The more I put dialysis behind me the more I began to move forward.

My faith was so strong, I began to lay hands on the dialysis machine and command it to bow to the name of Jesus. I would wave good-bye every time I would leave a treatment. A lot of the nurses may have thought I was just waving good-bye to everyone but I knew the Lord was going to bring me out one day. I began to spend most of my treatments reading my bible. I began to separate myself from everything that was not like Christ. This meant ungodly relationships and negative talk. I did not want anything in my life that was not Christ like. A lot of people thought I was weird but that was okay. There were young men trying to talk to me that did not understand about my lifestyle. That was fine I was comfortable being alone with my children and living holy. For the first time in my life I became content. I've always said, *dialysis was a blessing in disguise.* Not the illness, but it is where I truly received the Lord for myself.

After my first few treatments, I observed a younger patient. She was sitting directly across from me. I introduced myself. She said, *"her name was Nanette."* I told her my name was *Florence.* She was a few years younger then me. I also noticed she was stringing her own hemodialysis machine. I really admired her courage. I was curious about how she started being a self-care patient. I asked her, *"how did she learn to string her own machine?"* She told me, *"the nurses trained her."* (Wow I thought to myself, hey I can do that too). I began to think this experience might not be as bad as it first seemed. A nurse came around to check my vitals. I asked the nurse about learning to string my own machine. The nurse told me I would have to change my schedule to the 6:30 am slot. I told her okay the earlier slot seemed to work great for me. This meant I could get to the dialysis unit early. I would be done with treatments before the break of day. *"I told her to sign me up right away."*

This goes back to what I've said all alone: *It is always about how we deal with what happens to us that matters, we have a choice.*

"Steps towards Acceptance"

Once I learned how to string the machine, the treatments became more manageable for me. I began to learn as much information I could about dialysis. After about a week of training, I mastered the technique of stringing my own machine, monitoring my blood pressure and charting my progress. I was officially ready to go back to my regular treatment schedule. It was about time. I wanted to learn more from my new friend Nanette. Making the decision to string my own machine was the second best decision I ever made. *Leaving my children's dad was the first.* From that moment on, I became really good at taking charge of my health. I knew then I was an overcomer.

"Enduring More than You've Imagined"

Hearing for the first time that you have to undergo dialysis treatments in order to live can be very disturbing news. The doctors seem to bombard you with the news all at once. What is even more terrifying you may not have a lot of time in most cases to let the news settle in before choosing a treatment.

Healthy people have actually said to me, *"they would rather die than go on dialysis."* But I realize they would respond much differently if faced with no other choice, in wanting to live.

We are all unique humans beings that can live with more than we could ever imagine. It reminds me of a message I heard on a radio broadcast many years ago;

The speaker said, *be careful of how we view the person that robbed the 7-11, we don't know what drove him or her to that state of mind. The only thing that separates us from the robber is that we have not become desperate enough to do what they did—Author Unknown*

We don't know the desperation which drove the person to act. We never know how we'll react in any given situation. I know there is no way I could have seen myself doing any of the things I'm doing right now. Writing a book years ago was not something I would have foreseen in my future. Not to say that it wasn't a possibility. When I was first approached about the idea over ten years ago, it seemed almost hilarious to me. To me writing books was something people on television did, not common ordinary people like myself. My other reluctance about the idea was a weird feeling of knowing others would be reading my private thoughts.

There are certain things in life we have to face no matter what; *it is unavoidable.* A lot of times we are frightened when we are faced with what we don't understand. The other thing that frightens us even more are the horror story experiences of others.

Everyone does not view dialysis the same way that is why we have to be careful who we ask. You might even know of someone that died while receiving dialysis treatments. It doesn't mean they died because of the treatments. In some cases there are other conditions the patient could have been battling with. Uncontrolled Diabetes can be another factor that can cause complications with treatments. There were a lot of patients I dialysised with, who suffered with various other conditions in addition to ESRD. In most cases the complications from the other conditions led to the development of ESRD. Some of these conditions may include the following:

- Uncontrolled Hypertension
- Abuse of Pain Pills (Motrin, Aspirin)
- Uncontrolled Diabetes
- Infection
- Sudden Acute or Chronic Renal Failure
- Lupus

Some of these other conditions may have gone untreated or simply avoided. The abuse of any condition can be just as fatal as ESRD. There are issues we don't want to face about ourselves. Sometimes we don't take care of our bodies the way we should. We don't always eat all the right foods; we lack exercise or some patients abuse pain pills, cigarettes, street drugs and alcohol. In other cases there are patients who won't take medications the way they're prescribed. The effects of our behaviors don't always show up right away. Over time patients began to see the results of their behaviors down the road. In most cases the affects are often discovered when it is too late and in most cases the results are irreversible.

I can remember a patient that use to skip hemodialysis treatments on a habitual basis. In the beginning there were no immediate affects, but overtime the patient began to periodically pass out while undergoing treatments and had to be rushed in an ambulance to emergency. I thought after a few times of passing out it would be a wake up call. However the behavior did not stop. The patient was also diabetic. The patient refused to monitor the diabetes and eventually had to have a leg amputation. Missing treatments in addition to uncontrolled diabetes led to further complications. ESRD and diabetes can both be very complicated conditions to live with. Lack of self-discipline can be deadly in both cases. This went on quite a few years until eventually the patient passed away. It was a tragic loss for all of us that knew the patient well.

There are adversities we experience in our lives that we blame on the devil. While deep down we have helped the devil out many times over. Well there is no reason for us to get stuck there. What we have to focus on now is getting out of the mess we're in. Feeling guilty about how we got stuck in a situation is not going the deliver us out of it. That is why I am so thankful for God's Grace and Mercy. His Grace and Mercy is new every morning. He is a loving, kind and giving God.

(John 3:16 a) says, *for God so loved the world that he Gave His only begotten son.*

The Lord will deliver us in spite of ourselves. *Oh how I love Him, His love and kindness is better than life itself.* He knows just what we need. He will deliver us.

No matter what you're going through you hang in there. Help is on the way! To me it's never a question of if, but a matter of when?

He tells us in the book of Matthew that first things are first and that is: *But seek ye first the kingdom of God, and His righteousness; and all these things shall be added unto you* (Matt. 6:33).

What is it that you need from the Lord? The Lord has no problem blessing you, He's just waiting on you to get into agreement with His Word. Get to know Him for yourself. It is encouraging to know, He has healed others but it is a blessing to know that He will heal you too. While I was undergoing treatments it was a blessing to see others delivered. Their healing only solidified me seeing myself healed. You have to see yourself free and delivered. I hope that you will be richly blessed in the pages that follow. Most importantly don't expect God to do any less for you. (Eph. 3:20) says, *Now unto Him who's able to do exceedingly, abundantly above all that we could ask or think according to the power at work in us.*

Just imagine for a moment, He will not only heal your body He will also do far exceed anything you could ever imagine or what you could ever expect. He is going to do some things for you that you cannot even conceive into your thoughts. I don't know what this means to you but for me to even think about having the God of all creation living inside of me and working on my behalf is hard to even contain.

This only leads me to (Ish. 55: 8-9) where He says, *For my thoughts are not your thoughts neither His ways are our ways. Saith the Lord.*

The Prophet (Jeremiah 29:11) goes on to say, *For I know the thoughts that I think towards you saith the Lord. They are thoughts of peace, and not evil to give you an expected end.*

In other words we might be only thinking on the Lord healing us physically and He is looking at the whole picture. He sees us being totally delivered from everything weighing us down in life. Just knowing He has an expected end; that is only for the good of you and me makes me want to shout right now! Why wait until the battle is over shout now? Isn't it great to know we've already won the war? He's letting us know we are going to win!!

"You will not always feel His Presence"

While undergoing treatments there are times you will not feel up to being around anyone. A lot of times you might even close yourself off from the world. At times you'll become just plain irritated and annoyed with how you feel. People get tired of hearing about dialysis or that you're not feeling well today. In fact people can be down right insensitive. Therefore a lot of times ESRD patients learn to suffer in silence. It will be hard to express your feelings at times. Even if you do express your pain to others they can't help you anyways. Because of the condition you never know how you're going to feel. It is important to have your own space.

You need a place you can go regroup and collect your thoughts. In times like these meditate on the Word of God. The treatments are so unpredictable from one moment to the next. This has been my experience with the kidney transplant as well as being on dialysis. In one instant you have a machine dictating how you will feel while on the other hand you're taking anti-rejection drugs dictating how you will feel. This is why a Nephrologist will always say, *the kidney transplant is another form of treatment not a cure.* Either way there is just days you don't feel like being bothered. You don't even have to be going through any form of treatment to feel this way. This is a part of life.

In spite of each treatment I've tried, the kidney transplant is the best form of treatment available. *"You never knew how sick you really were until you receive a kidney transplant."* When you're going through the treatments you become immune to feeling a certain way. You don't even realize you have been sick for years. But once the transplanted organ is placed inside of you; it is simply indescribable.

I will never forget my first transplant: *When I woke up from surgery for the first time I was surprised to discover I began to feel better almost instantly. I thought it would be a while before regaining my strength, but much to my surprise it was almost instantly. My skin, hair, physical strength and memory started to return immediately. There is nothing that can replace a healthy organ. I don't care what anyone says, it's the best thing around.*

There are two things to bear in mind from my experiences. First all, *I have not only survived through the surgery once but twice.* Secondly, *I have been fortunate to not only to experience the cadaver-transplanted organ but also a living related donated organ.* There have been advantages and disadvantages to both. The table on the next page shows ESRD patients what to consider when choosing either type of transplant:

Organ Transplant	Advantages	Disadvantages
Cadaver	Patients are Free from dialysis. Patient can immediately receive transplanted organ once it arrives. Some patients may have the transplanted organ anywhere from 8 to 20 years. There are some patients that have the organ even longer (Each patient is different in how their body reacts)	There can be a long wait on the cadaver organ to become available. The wait can be anywhere from 3-7 years. Some patients die waiting for an organ When organ becomes available elevated antibodies can cause patients to be passed up on receiving a cadaver organ transplant. Organ life expectancy can range from 4 to 8 years. There is a possibility that the organ may not last a lifetime. Patient can have reactions to anti-rejection meds (all patients respond differently in the affects of medications) Patient will have to take anti rejection meds daily for the rest of their life. Sometimes even perfect matches won't work.
Related	Patient is Free from dialysis. Recipient has more of an advantage with the related organ lasting longer.	Hard to get related donors to donate organs. Sometimes even perfect matches won't work. Reactions to anti rejection meds

	Patients can feel a lot stronger. Even a related organ with one antigen that matches can last longer than a cadaver organ with all six antigens that match. Patients can get any where from 20 years to life with a related organ	Have to take anti rejection meds daily for life

Most patients don't have a variety of options in the type of organ that is available to them. Some patients only have the choice of receiving a cadaver organ.

While I was waiting for a cadaver organ, I spoke with another hemodialysis patient who had experienced a cadaver kidney transplant operation. One transplant patient said, *"her transplanted organ lasted only one day."* She went on to say," *if she had the opportunity to receive another cadaver kidney transplant again she would do so without any hesitation. Because that one-day was the best day of her life. Receiving the kidney transplant, was the first time in a long time she felt healthy again."* There is nothing that can replace good health. Therefore any type of organ is truly a blessing from God. This patient's reaction about the transplant only increased my faith. This only solidified my belief in having the transplant.

*It is my sincere hope for patients in waiting would read You're the Lord that Healeth...*and be challenged to see the Lord as a Healer in their lives. Please grab hold of what is rightfully yours, Jesus suffered thirty-nine stripes for you and me to receive this right. *Stand and Be Blessed!*

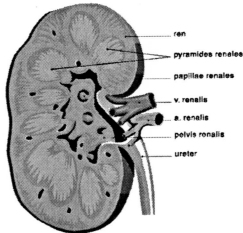

Photograph of a Normal healthy functioning kidney. For a normal healthy functioning kidney your blood passes through the kidneys 300 times a day. The nephrons clean all your blood in 45 minutes. Every day the nephrons send about six cups of urine to the bladder. -Information and Kidney Photograph Retrieved from ww2.saturn.stpaul.k12.mn.us/ki...

3
Adjusting To A New Way Of Being

I Beseech you therefore brethren, by the mercies of God, that ye present your bodies a living sacrifice, holy, acceptable unto God, which is your reasonable service (Rom. 12:1).

How one adjusts to changes in their lives is different for each individual. Being stricken with Glomeronephritis *(also known as End Stage Renal Disease)* is a progressive disease, which deteriorates the patient's renal function over time. The more advanced stages require some form of dialysis treatments or a kidney transplant. Without dialysis or a kidney transplant an ESRD patient will die.

"Serving A Purpose"

Everything in our lives serves a purpose. Our kidneys serve a very important purpose. *The Kidneys are the most vital organs in the body. The kidneys primary function is to cleanse all the poisons from the bloodstream.* **Dialysis** is a treatment which acts as an artificial kidney to do what the native kidneys can no longer do. The only limitation to the dialysis is that, there is no real comparison to normal healthy kidneys. Normal healthy kidneys are use to working 24 hours seven days a week. *The artificial kidney* is a dialyzer (plastic tube) used to administer a dialysate solution. The dialysate solution cleanses all of the blood in about 12-15 hours. The hours are generally done throughout a weekly process. The process is often divided into 3-day intervals. Although, the patient is able to function and live a normal life, dialysis does not give the total clearance a healthy kidney does. Patients can live well and long on dialysis. However, there is no compensation for the real thing. Another side effect of the treatments is, the damage that the body sustains. There is a lot of bone damage and damage to other organs. A lot of these damage is often irreversible. The process is not an easy concept to grasp for most patients. However, the sooner an ESRD patient accepts the process the better they will manage with undergoing treatments.

My late friend Ernie Wright a twenty-year hemodialysis veteran/former transplant patient referred to hemodialysis as a *"Prison Without Bars."* He felt that dialysis could be interpreted in three ways. First, *He says that you're sentenced to serving until your time is up.* Next, *he says that it can be like a dormitory.* There are some patients that make the treatments seem like home. Finally, *he said that it could be compared to a job. You're going to be there, the same place and time each week.* The way a patient interprets the treatment, is up to them. The only unfortunate thing is that it has to be done, no matter how the patient interprets the experience. Once you've reached the final stages of renal failure you have to receive some form of treatment in order to remain alive. I never say renal failure is not reversible. Because I believe God can do anything but fail. There have been patients that have gotten off of dialysis. It is not my attempt to build false hope. All things are possible to them who believe. No matter what stage you're in doing the progression of kidney loss, your internalization of what happens is the ultimate test of your faith.

Terry Clark a Hurley RDC dialysis social worker said it best, *"Patients that manage well on dialysis tell themselves they're not living for dialysis, but because of it."*

"Living with loss and discouragement"

What I regret most is the loss of friends who died prematurely from this disease. What saddens me the most, is a few of them died from giving up. They no longer wanted to live this way. There were a lot of patients I knew personally, that stopped going to treatments. Sure there are times I've gotten tired of going to one more treatment. During these trying times I'm often reminded of one songwriter who once said *"What a difference a day makes, twenty four little hours. "* There are times we have to just encourage ourselves. There have been nights I've laid hands on myself and said, *Florence you're going to make it through the night.* Even though I might be feeling really bad right then, I could not be moved by my feelings. Believe it or not, these words really helped me. Saying them out loud lets the enemy know, you believe God is in control.

If a song or my words don't remind me of how blessed I am, I turn to the Word of God. In (Psm. 30:5 b) David says; *weeping may endure for a night but joy cometh in the morning.* Wait until the morning comes. You've gone this long, what is another day?

A lot of things ESRD patients experience can make them become discouraged. In (Roms. 12:2a) Paul lets us know that *we are not to be conformed to this world: but be ye transformed by the renewing of our minds.* We have to renew our minds in the word daily. A lot of things would happen at the treatments which really upset me. If it was not for the word, I would not have made it through.

There were times I really was fed up with the nurse's continuously infiltrating my fistula site. After the first eleven months of being on hemodialysis, my fistula infiltrated during one of the treatments. I had to undergo emergency surgery to have it replaced. I had the fistula replaced with a graft.
A graft is a surgical connection of an artery and a vein with an artificial tube. The artificial tube will be used for the administration of dialystate solution during hemodialysis.

It seemed like every year, I was back into surgery for another replacement. Not to mention I had to have aneurisms removed. The aneurisms developed from the continuous overuse of the graft site. With each treatment the nurses are suppose to alternate the graft site. Alternation of the site will prolong the life of the patients graft.

Once the graft site is blown the patient has to go back into emergency surgery for another replacement. Now this process in itself can be very frustrating, especially since in my case I was running out of veins for the surgeons. Soon I knew they would have to place a graft in my leg. Fortunately, that has never happened. Making these types of adjustments can be the worst of times. After a graft is blown there's a six-week waiting period to allow the site to heal. A patient in the meantime has to still receive treatments. While I waited for the site to heal, I had to have a perma-catheter installed. *The catheter was inserted into a vein in my upper right chest area. The catheter had to be used in order for the treatments to be administered.* Even in the bad times I learned to call upon the name of Jesus. There are times I'm not always good with quoting scriptures. All I can do at those times is say the name of Jesus. There is power in the name of Jesus.

I could not imagine my two children growing up without me. There were so many times I didn't feel well. Just the thought of not being around for them was scary for me. Undergoing

35

dialysis can be very lonesome. It seems like no one understands. That is why it is important to have God as the center of your joy. Death can be all around you, yet He will keep you in perfect peace (If your mind is stayed on Him). It's okay to be frightened at times. But I always keep a word in the midst of the storm. Having the word hidden in my heart carries me over to the other side of the fear. I see what it means when (Psalms 119:11) says, *"Your word have I hidden in my heart that I may not sin against thee."*

I have also discovered that humming an old hymn is very comforting for me. There are a lot of times I sing an old hymn that says, *I'm so glad that troubles don't last always.* Singing will keep you when you're going through the rough times. The rough times will come but a song will harness your spirit by anchoring you, in knowing God has it all in control. I don't care what the enemy throws your way; with the Lord on your side you'll bulldoze your way through it. I can say that because I am here today because of praising Him in the rough times. A song kept me through the times I didn't think I would make it through. I don't know anyone that lives totally free from all trials and tribulations. In fact, I don't really care to be too sociable with people that have never experienced anything. People that have never experienced anything, tend to look down on what they don't understand. In spite of what we do, no one can control what happens to them. However, we all can choose how we handle what happens.

A fellow dialysis patient (the late Ernie Wright) further expressed in his article; *there are no vacation days from dialysis. There are no holidays, birthdays or whatever day that the treatments happen to fall on. Dialysis comes before your marriage, your kids or whatever is occurring at any given time.*

Dialysis does not care what events are going on in your life. You can do things you've always done but keeping them in proper prospective. Most of the time loved ones cannot understand why you're always irritable with them. Sometimes it even causes separation too. It is painful for me to watch how healthy people show such little regard for human life. They have no idea of how their lives can change in the twinkling of an eye. Dialysis can dictate how you'll feel physically on a routine basis. Contrary to how people would have you to feel.

I have learned that whatever is going on in my life at the present time, I cannot allow it to determine the final outcome. I am determined come hell or high water God has the last word. In spite of what any report says. I am going to fight ESRD with everything I got. Never loosing sight of the fact I have an enemy that is trying to kill me. This is my life and I have to fight with every fiber of my being. The Devil knows his job; he is always waiting for us to slip up on our end. Sure as I sit watching the blinking lights on the dialysis machine waiting for my time to be up, it is not always the most trilling experience of my life.

Therefore, during each treatment I have learned to make the most of my time. There are days I bring my bible and other inspirational books to read. If I am not in a reading mood that day, I will bring my tape recorder. I love to listen to praise music or a word filled life-changing message. There are days I don't feel like listening to a tape or reading. These times I find myself in a mood to sketch a drawing. Now these are things that work for me. Whatever you do to pass the time then you do that. These things help me to pass the time and take my mind away from everything that is going on around me.

You can live well on dialysis, if you choose to; you do have a choice. If you don't choose to make the most of your time, you'll find yourself very frustrated every treatment. In order for you not to focus on what is going on, it is important to divert your attention away from everything. *The enemy would have you to focus so strongly on what is before of you, instead of what can be in front of you.* If you talk to people that are managing well on dialysis, they'll tell you they have to prioritize the treatments. The more that you allow the treatments to consume your life it will. You will find that focusing on the treatments will make you only feel sorry for yourself. Believe me no matter what you are enduring there is, *always someone else that is a lot worse off then you.*

A lot of times we cannot see the forest for the trees. Don't hang your head down and ever think this is the end of your life. I really don't like the term *End Stage Renal Disease.* Because it not the end, until God says it is. I don't care what the diagnosis is, it can change at any time. Therefore, a diagnosis doesn't mean a thing. A diagnosis can change just the way it appeared. I am concerned with what God's word says about me. This does not mean I ignore the symptoms. Before someone or something tells you not to begin or to stop treatments make sure that you're truly hearing from God. Never step out on just an intuition. The enemy is a liar and a deceiver too. God will deliver you. We have to make sure that we're truly hearing from the Lord. We don't want to hear part of what the Lord is showing us. While the rest we jump out in ourselves.

If your doctor has told you to start dialysis treatments, then that is what you do. Remember, *the Lord is the Healer of the body not you.* A doctor can administer treatments but he can't heal the body. Even if you lay hands on someone to be healed, you are not the healer. We can't do anything in and of ourselves. If the Lord has shown you your healing, stand on His Word. Never let His Word leave your sight. Always take heed of what (Hosea 4:6) says, *my children are destroyed for lack of knowledge.*

Shortly after I began hemodialysis the Lord showed me I would be delivered. He never showed me how or when. All I knew was that the Lord showed me I was going to be delivered. A lot of times the Lord shows us what is coming but we have to go through something to get there. What I learned throughout the years before my healing manifested, it is a process. Not to say there cannot be an instant miraculous healing. The Lord can do anything but fail. But mine was a process.

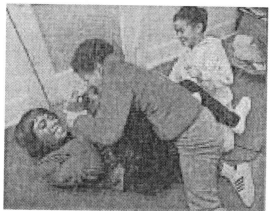

Photo taken by Flint Journal Photographer Stuart Bauer
(I'm Wrestling with my two children over candy)

4

Living With (ESRD)
End Stage Renal Disease

God is in control of everything. *Ye before the day was I am He and there is none that can deliver out of my hand I will work and who shall let it* (Isaiah. 43:13).

When I say living with ESRD, *"Living"* is a key word. I am living with ESRD, not merely existing. It grieves my heart for me to come across patients, who have told me that their lives were over. They lay in the bed day after day waiting to be served. There have been patients spouses that have asked me how can they get their husbands or wives back into life again? ESRD affects every patient differently. I believe how we deal with problems in our lives is how we will cope with ESRD. If every situation in your life is treated as a big catastrophe, that is how you will deal with ESRD. If you deal with situations like another challenge to conquer, that is how you will deal with ESRD.

39

"Living Life To The Fullest"

'*Life is what you make it.*' Life does not make you; you make your life. Everything you have become, started first with what you believed about yourself. If you believe that ESRD is the end of your life then it will be. But if you believe ESRD is something you can live with and overcome then you will.

I don't really think about ESRD until I go for a doctor's appointment or something that reminds me about dialysis. Other than that, I really never think about it at all. The best way to deal with the disease is not to make it the center of your life. When you do, it will affect everyone around you. I am not saying you won't have moments where you don't get depressed about how you feel. Just know that this too will pass. It always does and it always will. How you feel in one moment will change in the next few seconds. Our feelings are so fickle. Everything in your life cannot be based on how you feel. There are days I have taken a treatment and felt just like crap. I did not think I would be able to make it through the night. I woke up the next morning and felt great. This is why we can't base anything on how we feel.

I have learned the best way for me to cope with ESRD, is to find something I enjoy doing. You will be amazed how a great hobby will take your mind off of yourself. Think about starting one thing you've always wanted to do. It does not have to be a big thing, but one thing. *"Any Journey starts out one step at a time."*

Not to digress from my experience but I can remember when my husband and I started preparing his first book of poems. We did not know what was going to happen. But we started imputing one, two and three poems a day. Before long we would input about ten poems a day. After a while we would increase the input to twenty poems a day. Soon we were compiling volumes of poems. But we started out one poem at a time. Everything did not happen overnight. Nothing worth having comes in one night. If you gain instant success at anything and it came overnight it won't last. I always feel that anything worth having will always cost you something. In fact, it may cost you everything. Everything in my life came with a great price. You never know what you have, until it has been tried and tested. It needs to be tried in the fire.

When you look at someone doing well at something you're not, then it is something they're doing you're not. It is not that they have some sort of magic potion you don't. It is only they have the wisdom in the area you don't. Instead of thinking that they don't understand your situation, try to figure out why it doesn't matter. It doesn't matter how much money they might have. Just like a disease has no special preference on who it will strike worse. It is how a person has chosen to deal with the disease. A successful ESRD patient has discovered, *"dialysis is only a fraction of their lives."* I never saw myself on dialysis for the rest of my life. I felt from day one the Lord was going to heal my body. I did not know how or when but I knew, *"dialysis was only but a light thing for God."*

Healing comes in many forms. A lot of ESRD patients do not see a kidney transplant as a form of healing. But every good and perfect gift comes from above. Although a surgeon operates on a patient they cannot heal the body. The surgeon is just an instrument God uses to perform His miracles. Regardless, of the awesome gift that they have for performing such an extraordinary act, God is the Healer! This is why surgeons can never guarantee the outcome. All they know is that if everything is attached correctly it is suppose to function properly. Once it is attached they have to wait on the Lord to do the work. God uses the surgeon, to produce healing to the body. Anything that comes into the earth needs a willing vessel (a body). Good and evil has to have a willing vessel (a body) in order to operate.

You might ask what made me feel like I was somebody special? First of all, I know that I am a child of the King. Secondly, I knew I had more work to do for His kingdom. Finally, all of the things the Lord was showing me were impossible to do if I remained confined to dialysis. It would require me to perform at my best. I knew if the Lord was going to bless me and make me a blessing to people; I had to be delivered in order to do so. How could I be an effective witness, if I was still sick myself? It would be very difficult to profess God as a Healer, if I was not healed. People tend to turn away from a person that doesn't have a manifestation in their own lives. That only makes since.

In spite of it all, I continued to cry out to the Lord for my deliverance. He led me to (Mark 14:36a) *And (Jesus) He said, Ab'Ba Father all things are possible unto thee.* That is when I received the conformation my deliverance was on the way.

I began to see myself healed when I was undergoing treatments. A pastor I have known and admired for years told me I had to develop crazy faith in order to receive my deliverance.

He said, *"when everything in your life is saying the opposite of what the word of God is saying, in fact it seems like all hell is breaking loose; that is a confirmation your deliverance is on the way." Stand Still and Wait on the Lord.*

This advice seemed to match everything that was going haywire in my life right then. It seemed like once I got on with my life everyone would be happy for me. But instead people were treating me even worst.

In September 1992

I decided it was the right time to return back to school. I had been on dialysis for over a year. I decided if I returned back to school, I would not attend University of Michigan any longer. With my present condition, I felt more comfortable attending a smaller college that was more attentive to my needs. Being at a large University would require me to do a lot of walking. There were days it would be difficult to do so.

Ross Medical Education Center was running lot of advertisements for their Medical Assistant program. For me becoming a licensed Medical Assistant in less than a year sounded very appealing. Usually it takes two years to get licensed. I knew a few friends who graduated from the Ross Program. Ross took students through the course at a much faster pace then the other colleges. However, all I knew is I wanted to be an MA. Eventually, I shared my dream with one of the nurses at the dialysis unit. She told me she knew I could do it and she believed in me. She even promised to help me study at each treatment. After our talk I went and registered for the classes. The program was great but there was a lot of information to remember. My mother was very proud of me and glad to see me getting on with my life.

While I was attending classes, I began to see less and less of my mom. Between my studies, the treatments, and my children all my time was filled. It seemed like I would see my mom only when it was time to pick up the kids after treatments or in between leaving for classes. I would call her on the phone and apologize for not having a lot of time. She would say, *oh don't worry about it; just bring me some of those A's.* Little did I know that was going to be the last year I'd spend with my mom. Had I known; I would have spent every waking moment with her. When I look back on it now, the Lord was preparing me to get on with my life. After my moms death, I became consumed with my medical studies.

I believe that if I did not have the medical schooling at the time of her death, losing her would have been even harder for me to deal with. The loss of my mom was the fuel that drove me to achieve my goals. It was my desire to one-day work in the Pediatrics field. I was given the opportunity to do my externship, in the after Hours Pediatrics Clinic at Hurley Medical Center. I graduated from the Medical program with straight A's. I was also selected to give the speech at the graduation.

Once I became a license MA, some of the other hemodialysis patients seemed to become intimidated by me. There were patients that actually told me, I thought I was better because I didn't act sick. This couldn't be further from the truth. There were times I felt bad but I had learned to get back up and keep going. I'm not a person who shows my pain outwardly. I was astonished by the other patient's resentment. With my mother gone and having no friends, I felt very lonely. However, I continued to stand and believe the Word of God. I knew He was going to deliver me. The more ostracized I felt by other patients, drove me to the Word of God. One scripture in particular stood out to me during this time. The great King Solomon wrote in: (Ecc.1: 18) *For in much wisdom, is much grief.* The other scripture that I can relate to is (Job 42:2) which says, *I know that thou canst do everything and that no thought can be withholden from thee.* God is Omnipresent He is always available no matter what we are enduring. I continued to go to treatments, work part-time and attend Bible College. It gave me very little time to concern myself with other thoughts. There was a responsibility I had to my children. They needed to see that no matter what happens in life, we are resilient human beings that can still succeed.

There is nothing impossible for God to solve. (Luke 1:37) says, *For with God nothing shall be impossible.* I truly believe that every word of God is true. His word has been real in my life.

It doesn't matter what you're going through, He already knows. All you have to do is, call on Him. There is nothing too hard for Him to do. He just wants us to reach out to Him. He is patiently waiting with open arms.
(Jer. 32:17, 27) says, *Ah Lord God behold thou has made the heavens and the earth by thou great power and stretched out arms and there is nothing too hard for thee. Behold I am the Lord the God of all flesh is there anything too hard for Me?*

ESRD is a small thing to God. When we reach out in faith and only believe; there is nothing He won't do for us. There is nothing in this life we can't overcome. We have to only trust and believe never wavering in our faith.

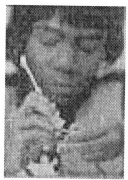

Florence (Phillips) Dyer age 30, stringing hemodialysis machine and administering Epogen injections into the lines. Photo taken April 1995 by Stuart Bauer/Flint Journal Photographer

5

Accepting the Condition

A sound heart is the life of the flesh; but envy the rottenness of the bones (Prov.14:30).

It is about time to listen to your body. There is no way around it. But you're the only one that can come to terms with what is going on. I discovered the more I learned about the dialysis treatments, the better I managed the disease. Patients do better when they learn all the things to look out for. Now that doesn't mean that patients who do well, have always followed everything to the letter. It doesn't matter which treatment you choose you're not going to always do everything perfect. There are holidays you're going to go overboard but learn to cut back afterwards. Whatever you do, as long as it is done in moderation you should be fine. It is when we abuse the wrong foods on a regular basis, day in and out that we get into trouble.

This is why it is important to listen to your body. If you don't, it will make you pay attention. There are a lot of patients that suffer from lots of cramping, do to overloads of food or fluid intake. Cramping can be caused by an ongoing cycle of overeating or too much fluid intake. It is important to be careful in either case. I had experienced some cramping on occasions, when I had to pull

45

off too much fluid. The cramping can be extremely painful. After a few times of experiencing these episodes, I had to make the decision to monitor my fluid intake. After experiencing enough situations like this, I eventually open my eyes. Unfortunately, a lot of patients I know have never learned this lesson. It is not easy to stay on the strict diet, hemodialysis demands from you.

"Taking Charge Of Your Health"

Hemodialysis requires a lot of self-discipline. Although, the dialysis machine cleanses the blood the patient has to work in conjunction with the machine. Working against the machine, is going to do more harm then good. Some patients returned home and piled on big plates of salty foods, for the next couple of days. Then the patient returns back to the unit the following day overloaded. This only causes the machine to work harder, to cleanse all the extra waste out of the bloodstream. This type of behavior is what causes cramping. In addition, to more damage to your body. All the machine knows is that it is designed to remove waste. It does not think about how much discomfort the patient might be in with the extra waste removal. It is time for you to accept your kidneys can no longer do what they once did. Even though dialysis is designed to remove the waste products there is no substitute for the real thing. Now a lot of this is easily said then done. I know for sure because I am a person that loves to eat. When I say love to eat, I really enjoy high rich foods. This is why I had to discipline myself to stop eating high rich foods like ham, pizza, and Chinese dishes. If you also have cravings to eat these types foods, then it is time to consider eating only a small portion. Personally, I knew if I did not eat what I liked then I'd wait until I became frustrated and eat more of it. Therefore, it is best to eat a portion then overindulge on it later.

It takes a lot of self-control to really discipline your eating habits. You are the only one who has the power to say, *this is all I am going to eat and move on.* Physiologically, we are designed to do the opposite of what someone tells us we can't do. When a

46

person tells me I can't do something, the forbidden seems to become more appealing to me. However, if they had never said anything then I would not have ever thought about it. It is better to use a little reverse physiology, when giving out an ultimatum.

To me the best method of reverse physiology, is to show a person an alternative way of not doing something. This makes it more appealing, then to just out right saying no. This is why I always choose to eat in moderation. We're going to eat the foods anyways. Just because you're on dialysis you can live well. There are patients that still enjoy a lot of the same foods they use to before receiving their treatments. These patients are able to moderately eat rich foods and manage their treatments very well. I am one of them, that's why I know it can be done. However, it must be done in moderation. I feel if you are going to be going through any adversity, you might as well enjoy yourself in the process.

There is nothing like having to do something you don't enjoy. To top it all off, you have to eat only pasted foods too. There is nothing more depressing for me then to be restricted from something I enjoy. That's why I have chosen to enjoy every minute of my life. Whatever food choices you make, always know your own limit. Sometimes we tend to overdo it and that's how we get into trouble. It is no different with the abuse of foods. It is the abuse of foods, and medications that is unhealthy for us. Realize when you've had enough and stop. Whenever I see myself getting into trouble I've learned to stop. Sometimes I have not stopped right away. But other times trough prayer, I've been delivered.

If you lack control over your appetite, then occasionally splurging on rich foods might not be best thing for you. We all know ourselves and you know what you can and cannot take. Use Godly wisdom, in everything you choose. If you don't have wisdom in that area, ask the Lord to give you wisdom. He promised to give us wisdom and abraded not. There is nothing He will hold back from you. When I discuss what I've experienced, it does not mean I have always made the best choices. However, I'm here to let you know you can live and still enjoy life on dialysis.

Your life does not have to end because you have been stricken with this horrible disease. I will never tell you everything for me has always been a bed of roses. I've literally been through Hell and back. Although, I've been through I am still standing. I want to share the good and the bad, so nothing is left to imagination. I don't want to see any other renal patient make some of the mistakes I have made. I also don't want to see patients afraid of receiving a kidney-transplanted organ. I believe I've had an experience with every form of treatment for a reason. First of all, there is no way I could let other patients know they can make it through the treatment.

Next, *You're the Lord that Healeth...* has allowed me to open my life to the world. I believe it was not by accident I'm writing this book. Finally, even if this book only reaches one ESRD patient, it will be a blessing for me. If only one patient sees himself or herself healed, is an encouragement I've done my part. In any case writing this book has allowed me to release a lot of painful emotions that would have remained untold. It is very unhealthy to live with regrets of what we should have done, than knowing we've done all we could. I feel better knowing there's nothing left to do.

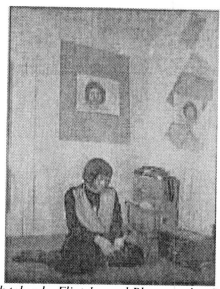

Photograph taken by Flint Journal Photographer Stuart Bauer
Listening to You're the Lord that Healeth Me

6

Living Life One Day At A Time

"Being on dialysis is only a fraction of who I am," "It's not all of me."- *Florence (Phillips) Dyer/Photograph taken by Flint Journal Photographer Stuart Bauer / Journal Staff Writer Rose Mary Reiz*
On November 4, 1993

My mother went to the doctor for a routine visit. To me there was no reason to be alarmed about anything. I was shocked, when I received a call from my cousin to rush over to the hospital immediately. The devastation in my cousin's voice was frightening enough. She told me my mom had lost consciousness. Upon my arrival to the hospital, I thought my mom would come around. I stayed the entire night at the hospital. My mom never regained consciousness. On November 5, 1993 my mother died from complications of emphysema and congestive heart failure. Her death came as a complete shock to my entire family. I was very angry about all the years doctors had not properly treated my mom.

She had suffered symptoms of renal failure that went misdiagnosis for years. My mother had experienced severe edema and was told to take water pills. Whenever I would try to talk to her about the similarity of her symptoms with my brother and I, she did not want to hear of it. It was not until towards the end of her life she was told about the development of kidney disease. Knowing my Mom, she could have always known about the kidney disease but did not want to share the diagnosis with me. This is something I will never know.

A couple days before my mom passed away, I had a horrible nightmare. In the nightmare, I dreamed my mom had died. The night I had the dream my children and I, spent the night with her. I was so frightened by the nightmare I jumped up out of the bed and rushed over to her side. I shook her really hard. She asked me, *what is your problem.* I told her, *oh nothing.* There was no way; *I would ever speak about my mom possibly dying.* I never wanted to ever consider the thought. My mom told me *she was dreaming I brought her a beautiful lavender dress. She looked at me with a smirk and said well I must have been dreaming, because you haven't bought me anything.* I said, *aw mom you're so crazy.* She dosed back to sleep. I left her house that day totally trying to forget the dream. To think about this happening was one of the most terrifying things I could ever imagine. Living with a kidney disease was not as terrifying as the thought of loosing my mom. Now I was faced with actually loosing her for real. Looking back on the dream now, I see it was a forewarning of what was going to happen.

All I knew was, it felt like someone had let all of the air out of my body. My mother was only forty-eight years old when she died. I could not believe one-day my mom was here and the next moment she was gone. How could I go on without my mom? For twenty-eight years of my life she was always there. Sure I had my children, my father, brothers and sisters, but no one could ever take the place of my mom. All my life she had always been there for me. Even though I have a lot of siblings we only get one mom that's all we get. It was hard to imagine the thought of going on without her. There were days, I could not see myself making it. But I did one day at a time. To this day I have never gotten over the loss but I have learned to live with it.

I believe we honor the ones we love that have crossed over by living our lives to the fullest. There were so many things my mom had never done in the forty-eight years of her life on earth.

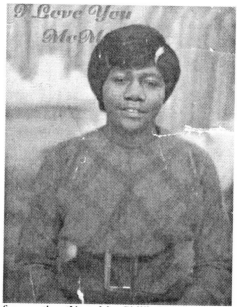

Photograph of my mother (Verta Mae Phillips) at the age of sixteen. She's posing in front of Niagara Falls. *(February 14, 1945- November 5, 1993)*

My mother never learned to drive a car. The photograph above is one of the very few photographs of my mother. She was never one who liked to take photographs. My mother has been gone almost eleven years now. It almost seems like yesterday she passed on to the other side. There is so much that has happened in my life since she died. I have so much I want to tell her. One day I will see her again. Because I know that those that die in the Lord are only resting from labor. She prepared me while she was here, that we all have to walk this way. There is just so much I want to say to her. I know a lot of momma's prayers have been answered and I am living the results of her prayers now.

While my mother was here, she always believed Floyd and I would receive a kidney transplant. Like most ESRD patients I was uncertain about taking that step. Obviously my mom knew me better, than I knew myself. My mother always told me, *I would be successful with my art. I could not have seen that either.* Now I am a successful designer. She said, *no matter what I did in life I would not be successful until I developed the gift the Lord gave me. It is okay if I pursue the medical field but God gave me a gift and that was my purpose in life.* My mother was right about that too. I am now living my dream and happier than I've ever been.

There were days her death was like a bad nightmare. I kept thinking things would be different once I woke up. I would wake up the next day and it was still real. Not only was it real I had to still go to hemodialysis. When I got to dialysis a lot of the nurses were watching my reaction. My mom seemed to be the only person that could keep me in line.

Now my mom was gone the nurses did not quite know what to expect. I was so depressed; I did not even feel like stringing the machine. I called in advance to make sure the nurses would have the machine strung before I arrived. Throughout the preparations for the funeral my sister came to sit with me at the treatments. I sat in my chair very quiet and distant. It was great having family around, but I knew it wouldn't last forever. Soon my sisters, brothers, aunts, uncle and my father would all have to return back to Chicago. But for now I would be able to enjoy them for the time they were here.

Once my family returned to their various homes, I had to face my mom was truly gone. How do you go on, when everything you have known in life is stripped away from you? It was difficult to get up and get going at times. But I did it anyways. My mother always was the one to talk to me about setting my priorities in order. I had lost my best friend. There was no one that could fill the emptiness I felt. My mother and I did everything together. She died around the thanksgiving holiday. We had just started putting together our thanksgiving dinner list. It was hard to even think about cooking. I was expecting my mom to walk through the door at any time. The first year of her death was the hardest year of my life. I spent the first holidays after my mom's death with various friends.

"Even in the hurt you will rise again"

For years because of my seizure disorder the doctors had banned me from driving. The ban was with a stipulation of remaining seizure free for up five years. Well that was one of the first things I decided it was time to be lifted. I had been seizure free for five years. During the time of my last seizure I was twenty-three and now I was twenty-eight. I spoke with the doctors about clearing me to drive. After several test the doctors decided I had been seizure free and it was time for me to go for my license. I passed the road test through *Sears Driving School.* I was so happy to be able to drive. I went out and bought a little inexpensive used car. All I thought about was if my mother could only see me now. But it still never took away the pain of her not being here with me. It was difficult to even drive down her street.

I continued undergoing treatments but it was like I was not even there. It was difficult for me to find a babysitter. My mom had always kept my children and I never trusted anyone else to watch my children. They had been to daycare when they were much younger. But I could not afford to pay what the daycares were asking for. For a while I had to bring my children with me to the treatments. The nurses were very understanding but it was very clear I had to come up with a better plan. After a couple babysitters I found the perfect sitter. Six months after my mother's death I completed my medical training and started working as a medical assistant a couple months after graduation. Everything began to look up for me again. Until my car eventually broke down and I had no way of getting to work. My dad was nice enough to give me a better car.

On November 15, 1994, I had a day off from work and my children were home from school. I decided to take the kids out for

53

a ride. We stopped at McDonalds to get some hamburgers and fries. While I was driving on the expressway, the children were acting up in the back seat. I began yelling at them to keep it down. They continued to keep up the commotion. After a while I decided to pull the car over to the shoulder of the expressway. Suddenly, I lost control over the wheel. The car tumbled over so fast. All I can remember was the car flipping over and over again. In the process of tumbling over, I began thinking we're all going to die! My daughter was frantically screaming and I could do nothing to save her, my son or myself. Suddenly, in the midst of us tumbling over there was a peace that came over me. It gave me an assurance we were going to be just fine. The car rolled over about five times. All at once the car came to a complete stop and we were all stuck upside down.

Until this day, I cannot explain what happened. All I know is an angel saved us that day. My son kicked the door open and there was a man helping us out of the car. It was as if the Lord had a rescue plan right there waiting for us. The ambulance and the police came right away. The police officer said, *that we were lucky to be alive.* After being examined at the hospitals the doctors decided to keep me overnight for observation. My children were sent home with relatives.

My doctor ran additional test, to see if I had a seizure. If I did have a seizure they could revoke my license. The test showed there had not been any recent seizure activity. I was cleared to continue driving. After returning home for a while, it was difficult for me to think about ever driving again. I felt so bad that my dad had given me such a nice car and I totaled it out. What gave me great consolation was, being blessed with our lives. We could replace the car but we could never replace us. A few months after the accident I bought another car. Although I felt comfortable driving, it took me a long time to get back up on the expressway again. However, I don't think the children trusted my driving for on the expressway for a while either.

Eventually, it was unavoidable. It came a time I had to tackle my fear of driving on the expressway again. My brother

Frank needed a ride to work one day. Unfortunately, the only way to get to his job was by using the expressway. He placed me in a position where I could not say no. If the expressway driving was not bad enough, my brother worked an hour away. Therefore, you can only imagine the hesitation that went through my mind. Either way he had to get to work and no way there. I decided to say yes. My brother drove on the way there and encouraged me I would be fine on the way back. The only thing I kept thinking of the whole time he was driving, was that I had to drive back. If the driving wasn't enough anxiety my children were with me again. I was frightened about the possibility of getting into another accident.

Once we arrived at my brother's job it was my turn to drive back home. He told me *Florence you can do it, I know you can.* It was great to know he had more confidence in me then I had in myself. When I think back on it now, it was the Lord who set me up again. Once I began driving, I turned up the volume on the radio, so that praise and worship music completely filled the atmosphere. Once I began to mediate on the music soon I was able to relax. The Holy Spirit reminded me about all the Lord had brought me through. It wasn't before long after this day I was using the expressway again on a regular basis. I felt blessed to be alive and to taking charge of my life again. I believe that a lot of the blessings were being released in my life, because of my mother's prayers.

All that the Lord had brought me through suddenly began to increase my faith even more. It was as if a peace was resting over my life and I began to feel that everything was going to be just fine. It was still hard to imagine myself living without my mother but I had to keep going. There were two young impressionable lives depending on me. The Lord began to raise me up in all areas of my life. I began working hard and enjoying life again. Reading the bible became more and more of my daily nutrition. The dialysis treatment days seem to be the best time for me to get really deep into the word. Through reading the word, I began to discover how God uses all kinds of ways to administer divine healing. I began to discover that healing could come through the natural remedies of medicine. Whatever medium the Lord administers healing, always remember that every good and perfect gift comes from above. Therefore, every form of healing comes from the Lord.

Sometimes we limit the way we will allow our blessings to flow. We tie the hands of God, when we won't consider any type medical intervention. Looking back I can remember the times I turned the doctors away. It was difficult making the adjustment to hemodialysis; it was frightening to even consider the transplant. Until one day while I was undergoing a treatment the Holy Spirit lead me to a scripture in (II King 7:3-7 Amplified) about the four men stricken with Leprosy.

The scripture says, *Now four men who were stricken lepers were at the entrance of the city's gate; and they said to one another. Why do we sit here until we die? If we say, we will enter the city-then famine is in the city, and we shall die there; and if we sit still here, we die also. So now come, let us go over to the army of the Syrians. If they spare us alive, we shall live; and if they kill us, we shall but die. So they arose in the twilight and went to the Syrian camp, but when they came to the edge of the camp, no man was there. For the Lord had made the Syrian army hear the noise of chariots and horses, the noise of a great army. The Syrians arose and fled in the twilight and left their tents, horses, donkeys, even the camp as it was, they fled for their lives.*

The lepers came to the conclusion; *no matter what they did or didn't do they were going to die.* I began to see myself in these scriptures. The Lord showed me I was living in fear. I began to see no matter what I did or didn't do I could die. He enlightened me to see, how I was so afraid of dying I'd rather sit there. Doing nothing was helping me to feel safe. But was I truly safe? The words kept gnawing at my spirit; *Why sit ye here until we die?* I would never know like the lepers what was behind the other door. If I never stepped out there, I would have never discovered my healing.

In order to receive something you've never had, you've got to do something that you've never done-unknown Author.

It was at that very moment I was totally delivered from the fear of worrying about dying. No, I did not want to die but I no longer worried about dying anymore. Death will happen and when it does there is not much we can do about it anyways. But the life changing moment for me was when I read, the one part of the scripture. That scripture still stands out in my mind *"Why sit ye here until I die."* I suddenly realized I could be out enjoying every minute of my freedom. That is when; *I officially got on the cadaver donor transplant list.*

It is now ten years later and I've often thought about if I would have handled things differently. When I think about it; no I wouldn't have. There is a time and a season for everything. Had I decided to do one thing differently in the wrong season things would have turned out much differently. God has perfect timing for everything. One thing done totally out of order will set us off on a totally different course.

I can remember the day the doctor called me about the cadaver organ. It was the most exciting and scariest day of my life. I wasn't scared about the surgery. I was more scared about how, I was going to feel afterwards. I had not been healthy since I was eighteen years old and I was now thirty. Oh I dreamed of being healthy. There were so many other patients I dialysised with that said, *there was no way they would ever get a kidney transplant or have a second kidney transplant.* This was not very encouraging words for me. Especially, since I was now considering the transplant.

One patient I remember suffered two heart attacks after his last rejection episode. He was back on hemodialysis and very adamantly said, *there was no way that he would ever be so stupid to go through another transplant again.* This is just one of the horror story experiences. Although he had valid reasons to feel this way, I could not allow this negativity into my spirit. These bad experiences can influence your choices, if you allow them too. While I was undergoing the transplant evaluation process I attended several transplant conferences. I had the opportunity to meet and get acquainted with a lot of successful transplant patients.

There was one guy that had his transplanted organ for over twenty-five years. I met another kidney transplant patient that had his kidney for seventeen years. This was very encouraging for me.

One thing that a couple of the patients at the conference experienced and they warned me about *was, the first call they received was from a doctor was not a very pleasant call. The doctor told the patient he might have a kidney available for them and later called back to tell them that the kidney did not match. I did not even want to think about this happening to me.* They did not want to share this information with me (especially since I was waiting on an organ). But they wanted me to be aware that this experience could happen to me. They said, if I did receive this type of call not be alarmed. They also received another call and it was their kidney.

There was also another young lady there that said this experience happened to her twice. When the 3rd call came in, *"she told the doctor that it better be a match or don't call her anymore."* Thank God that it was the one for her. She had received the kidney six years prior to attending the conference.

I've shared these experiences about these patients to say, just as there are horror stories there are just as many success stories too. Making a life changing choice to have a transplant requires patients to do all their homework. It is best to speak with both sides. I made it a point not to ignore the good or the bad. It is important that you pay attention to all sides. This is a decision that you don't go into half hazardly. Your choice for the transplant is going to be a life changing experience and one that you will live with the rest of your life. Being misinformed or under informed can have some very disappointing consequences later on. Never totally discard the bad because it can have a ring of truth that prepares you for what to watch out for once you receive the transplanted organ.

I needed to know and understand just what I was getting myself into. It was difficult enough adjusting my life to hemodialysis. Now I had to think about, adjusting to a serious operation and anti-rejection medications. I wanted to weigh the good and the bad. I didn't feel comfortable just letting the chips fall where they may. After attending the conference, I decided not to even think about it anymore. I thought that when it happens it will happen. But I was not going to live my life everyday waiting for it to happen. I received a pager while attending the conference. I had so much uncertainty as to what would ever come of the whole thing. One good thing is that I passed the transplant evaluation with flying colors.

My name was officially on the *Cadaver Organ Transplant List*. The only thing that made it seem like a shot in the dark was there were a lot of people ahead of me. I thought it might be a one in a million chance I would receive an organ so soon. I wasn't shocked at it happening, because it was not a question of if, just always a matter of when. The only thing I can say is that it will happen soon enough. Worrying or concerning yourself about it is the least of your problems.

Whenever I get into worry I have to remind myself when Jesus said; *take therefore no thought for the morrow; for the morrow shall take thought for the things of itself sufficient until the day is the evil thereof.* (Matt. 6:34)

It is important to deal with what we can now. Because right now is all we really have. We don't know what tomorrow may bring. All we can go by is what is before us now. I continued to live my life each day without the thought of how I would react to the news. I was so busy working a part-time job as a Medical Assistant. My children were in school fulltime and I had returned back to College. I was active singing in the church choir and taking care of my rebellious teenage brother. Believe me my plate was overflowing. I had enough to think about, I could not worry about when the organ would come.

On May 14, 1995

I attended my grandfather's funeral in Chicago. My grandfather was ninety-one years old when he died. He had been on hemodialysis for five years. Complications from *Congestive Heart Failure* lead to him developing ESRD. While I was on my way to Chicago I *said to myself well maybe I'll take the pager with me, who knows I might get a page about a kidney.* I said this kidding because no one had ever called before. At the time of the funeral I was left with no time to study for my final exams. I decided that my children and I would carpool with my other siblings to attend the funeral. I left my homework back in Flint and thought if was best to finish once I returned. Since we were not going to be staying very long, I thought I'd have enough time to complete my homework. We returned home about 11:15 pm on May 15. It was barely enough time to get anything done. The homework had to be turned in on May 16 by 10:00 am.

Studying for the exam turned out to be an all-nighter. After about 2:30 am on May 16, I decided to throw in the towel. I got up from the table and walked up the stars. I still had my pager hooked to my belt buckle. Once I unclamped the back snap the buzzer instantly went off. It stunned me for a moment because it had never gone off before. All I knew was that I was so tired and it was so late. I thought about what the other patients had shared about the first call for the kidney didn't match. Trying to avoid the page I continued to get ready for bed because I could barely keep my eyes open. Then the buzzer went off again.

I turned on the bedroom light and did not recognize the phone number. I picked up the telephone and dialed the number that was in the pager window. Dr. Schroeder's voice was on the other end of the phone. He said, *Florence I have been trying to page you. I think we have a perfect match for you.* I said, *Dr. Schroeder you paged me at 2:30 in the morning to tell me that you think you might have a perfect match for me?* (The thoughts immediately running through my mind reflected back to the other transplant patient's experience. They assured me not to worry if it was not my kidney).

Dr. Schroeder said, *he would call me back in about five minutes to confirm if they had a perfect match.* He told me to, *"stay by the phone just in case."* I said, *"okay."* (after hung up the phone, it was difficult trying to get over the initial shock of the phone call. Each minute seemed like an eternity).

About five minutes later he called me back to say, *it was a perfect match for me.* He went on to say, *"I know you might need a little time to get your children situated. But please try to get over to the hospital as soon as possible.* He said, *he'd meet me at the hospital as soon as he could."*

Dr. Schroeder began to notice; I was not saying anything the entire time. He then hesitated for a moment and said *"Florence I know that you want this kidney right? Don't you?"*

I said, *yes I do Dr. Schroeder I was just trying to digest the news that it is actually happening for me.*

Dr. Schroeder said, *"okay I'll meet you at the hospital you try to get there as soon as you can."* He also said *"that he is going to give the hospital a directive not to begin the surgery until he arrived."*

(After hanging up the phone) I immediately started making phone calls, to make sure my children were going to have a place to stay. I called their father and he claimed he could not keep the kids. Before dialing the number, I was already used to him not being available to help. He always refused to help, especially when I needed him the most. Never mind that I was about to have major surgery. Even though he refused to keep his children, I was not going to let him upset me. I knew that the enemy wanted me to get upset, by something I already knew.

Therefore, I called my cousin and she told me that she would keep the kids. She was complaining about it, but she knew I needed a babysitter. It was not easy trying to find someone that would keep them on such short notice. Most of what I have discovered is that people can be very selfish, when it is not their lives at stake. Never mind that it was a matter of life or death. This is what I mean when I've said that people can be very cruel. I dropped the children off at my cousins and drove myself straight to the hospital.

Once I arrived at the hospital, the transplant team had me lined up to undergo a battery of test. The tests were to make certain I was healthy enough to receive the organ. While I was being tested to see if my body was strong enough, the doctors were also testing the cadaver organ. Everything had to be in order before surgery.

"The Success of the Cadaver Kidney"

The surgery was very successful and I was discharged after six days. During my stay in the hospital, I met another transplant patient named Arthur. Arthur had received his organ one day before mine. We were able to comfort each other throughout the recovery process. We were able to swap stories about our experiences with hemodialysis and our new organ. I believe that our bonding really helped both of us to recover very soon. We exchanged phone numbers and kept in touch to share additional information. The recovery process went by very fast for both of us. During my recovery, I met a wonderful guy. It had been years since I had dated anyone. But my children adored him and I did too. A month after surgery it was time for me to return back to work. Although, it was a blessing to have the kidney, the bills had to still get paid.

A few months after the surgery, I was recommended for a fill-in position. I took it because I needed to make some extra money. It might seem ironic but I began working as a fill-in Medical Assistant, at a nearby Kidney Center. Working at the dialysis unit gave me an opportunity to be on both sides of dialysis. I had a chance to meet patients that were frightened like myself, (when I walked in for the first treatment years ago). A lot of the patients had received the same life changing report. Identifying with the patients from first hand experience was very rewarding for me. Although, I had only received the cadaver transplant for a short time, I was able to inspire hope for a lot of other patients. Working at the unit with my newfound health was still really frightening. *The thought of my life changing in an instant never left me.*

It had only been just a few months after receiving my transplant. There was some emotional discomfort I was struggling with. Always in the back of my mind, I was battling with how long it would all last. This was a battle I had never fought before. The previous battle of life changing events was all too familiar. It seems like every time I became too comfortable with my life there was always another transition; *I had to get use to again.* One of the counselors that I worked with thought, I was an excellent candidate to speak with all the new patients.

What I felt that the counselors did not understand was, there were a lot of demons I was wrestling with. In the back of your mind, you'll never get over the fact you can return back to dialysis at any time. Once you have been on dialysis and although you're away from it, this is a *truth* that you'll never get over. You'll learn to live with it, but you'll never get over it. It does not matter how many years has gone by, this never leaves you. Life is filled with so much uncertainty.

While I was working at the dialysis unit, I received a marriage proposal from the guy I was dating. He came into the unit one day and he asked me to marry him. It is evident that my answer was yes. He is now currently my husband. There was so much going on in my life at the time. Just a few months prior to my engagement I lost my grandfather to ESRD.

During the time I was working at the dialysis unit I was recommended for a new position. My dream position came through. It was a position working fulltime as a pediatrics MA. There was so much on my plate. I was receiving job offers, I had just received a cadaver kidney and now I had accepted a marriage proposal. There were so many blessings in my life it was so overwhelming. It was hard to contain it all. When the 3rd chapter of Malachi speaks about the Lord pouring out blessings, you won't have room enough to receive; this scripture is beyond comprehension.

When I was discussing wedding plans with my fiancée, it was unbelievable I would be getting married. For a long time, I was afraid to consider dating anyone. I thought no one would be able to understand ESRD. A lot of times, I thought it was best for me to be alone. I did not want my illness to be a burden on anyone.

After the break up with my children's father, just the thought of another relationship was frightening.

It was hard to imagine a young man would be able to look past the fact; my condition could change in an instant. With ESRD there is so much uncertainty. There was never anyone in my life that had developed a relationship with my children and me. But I felt sure he was the one.
On December 5, 1995

I became Mrs. Florence Juanita Dyer; after marrying the love of my life, Mr. Ted Alan Dyer. The Lord always gives us just what you need. Ted can be my greatest support; especially in my darkest times. He always has a poem or a word of encouragement to keep me going. Even though he can be my greatest support, there is only one that can satisfy the longing of the soul. Nothing can ever replace who the Lord is in your life. Everything outside of my relationship with the Lord is merely a reflection of His goodness. Having the support of family and friends is really a blessing. I've truly been blessed with Godly friends.

Not all of my friends have dealt with ESRD. In fact most of my friends are quite healthy. A lot of them have never undergone any serious health issues. They have all remained a strong shoulder to lean on. Michelle and her husband Norman Gurley have always been a great supportive couple and Godly friends.
I believe the Lord places a variety of friendships in our lives. These friends can be a great source of strength and encouragement. Michelle has always been there for me.

When I lost my mother Michelle always had an encouraging word for me. It was a time I felt so alone and needed a friend to talk to and she was there. She was there for me throughout my sickness and the transplant too. Even during the time I got married she was there to comfort me and give me great advice. It is important to always appreciate those great friendships in your life. Although we don't speak on a regular basis I know she'll be there if I needed her. None of our friends are there by accident. Sure I've had a lot of takers in my life. But the Lord has placed a lot of givers in my life too. Throughout the years I have learned how to discern between the two.

I look at every person, place or thing as serving a purpose in my life. Either it is to make me stronger or to challenge me to grow. I don't only want people in my life that are only like me.

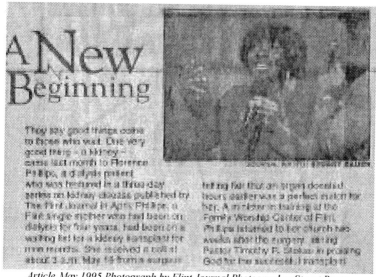

Article May 1995 Photograph by Flint Journal Photographer Stuart Bauer

7
The Gift Of Life Creates
"A New Beginning"

"All things come to those who wait," So they say. But there is waiting...and then there is waiting. –Flint Journal Staff Writer/Rose Mary Reiz

While waiting for a kidney transplant, you can use the time to achieve certain goals. The stress of waiting for a transplant organ can almost kill you. You're constantly planning for something that you don't know when it'll happen? You're wondering if it'll happen for you? And last but not least if you'll ever return to good health?

Being an African American the chances are very slim, of getting a perfect match. In addition to waiting most African Americans are not very generous donors. The Flint Journal ran a three-day article that featured three-kidney patients battle with hemodialysis, CAPD and receiving a kidney transplants. One of the articles featured was about my struggle with hemodialysis (the goal of the article was for raising awareness of the need for more organ donations).

The article ran one month prior to me receiving the cadaver kidney. The article generated such an enormous amount of feedback. There was a young lady named Cynthia, who was especially moved by the article. She contacted the Flint Journal and they directed her to the church where I worshipped. She was so moved by my story she felt compelled to contact me right away.

Once I spoke with the young lady, I was stunned by her offer. She said, *"she felt lead of the Lord to donate one of her kidneys to me."* I was almost speechless and did not know how to respond. There is no way I could have known the article would spark this type of a response. While talking with her the Lord dropped it into my spirit, to invite her to our church to worship with us. I was amazed by her generosity. She was so giving and kind and very compliant with the idea of attending the church with me. In fact, we met, worshipped and had the greatest time. I introduced her to my pastor and other members of the church. After worshipping together we made arrangements to meet with the transplant coordinator at Hurley. I thought wow this is my kidney. This was truly unbelievable.

We both met with the kidney transplant coordinator. The coordinator was not as impressed as I was. She asked to meet with me in private. Once we were alone in her office, she expressed why she had reservations about preceding further. She did not want me to get my hopes up too high. She was very apprehensive with the media coverage possibly being a motivation behind the young ladies generosity. She was not totally apposed to the possibility.

However, during the time we made the suggestion Hurley had never performed a *Living Unrelated Kidney Donor Transplant.* Another one of the coordinators major concerns was about, me being hurt down the road. Her final analysis of the situation was to wait. She said to wait about six months to see if the young lady was still interested in donating the organ. She felt that if she was still willing to donate by than we could take it to the board. I thought she must be crazy, that meant six more months of hemodialysis. However, I was willing to comply with proper procedures. Before I left, the transplant coordinators office she advised me *to view the situation as a sign from the Lord that my kidney was on the way.* A week later after meeting with the transplant coordinator my kidney was released.

"All Things Have A Purpose In Our Lives"

After having the kidney transplant the coordinator came to visit me in the hospital. The Transplant Coordinator and I both rejoiced over the blessing. She reminded me of the confirmation the Lord showed, through the young ladies generosity.

The Lord knows just how to get us to the place where we can receive from Him. The following year after, I received my cadaver kidney transplant the transplant coordinator contacted me. She said, another hemodialysis patient suggested an *Living Unrelated Kidney Donor Transplant.* She was excited that Hurley was about to perform their first unrelated kidney donor transplant. She said, when the idea came across her desk again she immediately thought about me. It is great to know I had a hand in opening the door for that possibility. The Lord used me to plant a seed in the heart of the transplant coordinator. Sure the young ladies kidney was not mine but just seeing a door opened for someone else was a blessing.

When we are going through a waiting process the Lord will send us confirmation to let us know the miracle we have been waiting for is on the way. The young lady only opened the door to let me know that miracles could happen for me. When I received the possibility that my kidney was not far off the Lord was able to release more blessings my way. We should *never despise humble beginnings.* Each level that we are on, the Lord has dealt to us the measure of faith. We have to open up our hearts to receive what he has for us. Faith is being promoted to another level in God. The Lord will meet us right where we are. That is why we should be ever increasing in faith. Every time we are delivered from one situation and transitioned into another state of being our faith should be much stronger. What was okay on one level will not work on another. The Lord has not changed but He wants us to know Him in a deeper way each time we are delivered out of each trial.

There are times we will remain in a place, until the Lord knows we are ready to move on. We're not delivered out of a situation until we get it right. We will continue to go around the same mountain, over and over again flunking the same test. When I first started hemodialysis, it wasn't the time for me to consider the transplant. There is no way I would have received the possibility of having one. God knows the right timing. He knows us better than we know ourselves. Not only does God know when we're ready, the enemy also knows when we're ready too. God's delays are not God's denials. Our timing is not always God's timing. Our timing is not always what is best for us either. I am so glad that my trust is totally in Him.

Two weeks after receiving the cadaver transplant, the Flint Journal featured a follow up story. The story was about me receiving the *Cadaver Kidney Transplant.* The article inspired hope for patients in waiting by demonstrating that, "*all things come to those who wait.*" I received my transplanted organ one month after the first article was featured. In fact, my wait on the donor list was nine months. It was a miracle I received a cadaver kidney so soon. Well I am here to tell you that it can happen for you too.

The first step is getting on the list. I realize that receiving my kidney that soon it was a blessing from the Lord to release the organ out of sequence. However, when the Lord wants to get a blessing to you He will leap over hills, mountains, valleys, or even part the red sea to do whatever it takes to get it over to you. There are times I still have to remind myself that the Lord skipped over thousands of patients to get to me. I always bear in mind that what God has for me it is for me. It is not to say that the Lord did not care for the other patients. (Luke 8:43-48) *talks about the multitude of people that were looked over for the woman with the issue of blood.* The woman's faith touched Jesus. It is important for you to know that it can happen for you. I am not trying to raise false hope, but I believe (Rom. 2:11) when it says that; *"There is no respectable person to God."* Therefore what He has done for others He will also do for you. You never know what is going to happen for you once you start believing. Be rest assured, if you are putting the word of God to work in your life; whatever you need from the Lord will come to pass. As long as it is in the will of God, it has to come to pass. (Num. 23:19) says that, *"God is not a Man that he should lie nor the sun of man that he should repent."* Therefore anything can happen if you only believe.

The average wait is 3-7 years. But I know that the Lord will skip over hills, mountains and reach down into the depths of the lowest valley to pull His children out. If you are a child of God you are no ordinary ESRD patient. Don't you fool yourself into thinking you're just like anyone else.

Although, we go into the fire, we don't go through the same way others do. Everything that happened to me happened very differently for other patients. Do I think that I am special? Yes, I am. Being a child of the King has its advantages. He promised never to leave us, nor to forsake us. He never said, we would not go through anything. No matter what comes against us in life, just knowing that the Lord is in control will give you the peace to stand. Always remember; *whatever doesn't kill you, can only make you stronger.*

I have counseled with a lot of patients waiting for an organ and others that were transplant recipients like myself. A lot of the recipients would agree with me when I say don't expect the transplanted organ to resolve all of your problems. The word says, *too much is given; much more is required of you.* There are some patients who are waiting for the transplanted organ to resolve pre-existing problems. They've forgotten that when their kidneys functioned normally they never resolved all their problems.

Some patients feel that once they get a kidney transplant-then they'll go back to school, return to work, get in shape or they will began doing things once again. They've set themselves up for a big shock. The information that I'm about to share with you is not meant to scare you but give you something to consider while you wait. There are no guarantees the transplanted organ you receive will function. Also if it does function there may be rejection episodes that can lead to failure. Your faced daily with the stress of endless possibilities you've never had before. The organ that you receive is almost like it has a mind of its own. The organ knows that you're not the native residence no matter if you are a perfect match; <u>he or she wants to leave!</u> The organ never gives up the fight for trying to escape from its new home.

The best implants can have delayed starts. The organ may even require that patients have additional dialysis treatments once the organ is transplanted. This does not mean there is anything to worry about. It is just every patient's body functions differently. The average cost for the transplant operation can range from $70,000 to $150,000 or more. Some insurance companies will cover most or all of cost for the operation but may vary from state to state.

This cost does not include extra expenses for lab work, rejection episodes. Rejection episodes can cost up to $10,000 depending upon how many episodes you're experiencing. Then there is the monthly cost for the anti-rejection medications. The cost of the anti-rejection medications can start at $2,000 or more monthly. The cost and dosage may vary based on the needs of the patients. The anti-rejection medications have to be taken daily for the rest of your life. I realize that a lot of this information may be a lot to digest right now. But I wanted to make sure that you were fully aware of the *Gift Of Life.* This is the point where I say it again; *to whom much is given much more is required.* I am not relating the information about the transplant to discourage you from getting one. I am merely trying to make sure that you are fully aware of the complete picture.

The information about the cost for the medications are extremely important. There are some insurance companies that will cover the cost of transplant medications for up to three years. It is important for patients to learn as much information about the medications before they're transplanted. If one dosage of the transplant medication is skipped the kidney can fail. Contrary to dialysis the organ brings with its own mysterious set of adjustments.

My life changed the moment the kidney was implanted. Unlike some organ implants, my kidney started working the moment it was attached. The transplanted organ since then has fought against some very impossible odds. I have found out since the transplant I am now on my own. While on hemodialysis it seemed like I received more emotional support. Sure there are support groups that I can attend now. But while on dialysis I had friends I saw three times a week. Now when I go to visit a lot of them either they are depressed or some have even passed on. It is very difficult finding a lot of transplanted patients that can relate to what I am experiencing. In addition to adjusting to the difference in my new life I learned that I had to change my eating habits again. First, imagine being restricted for four years, not allowed to exceed five glasses of water daily while on hemodialysis. I had to exclude certain fruits, foods or sodium products too. Once a surgeon releases you, he'll probably tell you to drink as much as you want.

The survival of the transplanted organ depends on how much water is imputed. Not drinking enough water can cause the kidney to dehydrate. Your bladder does not care what the organ wants. It is not ready to be overworked. The bladder has grown accustomed to not working for years. Now all of a sudden a foreign object is moving in and wants to run things. The bladder has had a good time doing as little work as possible. He is not about to let some crazy foreign object take up space and tell it what to do.

The organ also places demands that cause you discomfort. Any unexpected changes can lead to some devastating consequences. As of today, any decision you make or don't make compromises you keeping the transplanted organ. Therefore it is imperative that you keep it functioning for as long as possible.

The longer you're away from dialysis the stronger you feel. The more problems you experience with the transplanted kidney the scarier it seems. I don't care how long you're off of dialysis the effects of the experience stays with you. Every time you look at the scars you are reminded of where you've been. However every time you don't have to take a treatment you are encouraged about how far you've come.

I have endured three rejection episodes after my first year of receiving the cadaver kidney. I thank God I had not experienced another one during my second year. I suddenly got to the place where my third year went without any complications. In spite of it all, I had to endure I don't regret having the transplant.

I've experienced a few setbacks, but it has been worth every moment of my freedom. Now I have been given a second chance to be all that I can be. I have never met my donor family face to face. I've made contact with the donor family through cards and letters. I wanted to express my eternal gratitude. There are never enough words that can be said, for the gift they have given my family and me. I wanted them to know that their loved one did not die in vain. The family has written me back a couple of times. There is not a day that goes by I am able to forget that a person died and because of them I am enjoying the freedom I have today. I have some consolation that they did not die because of me. But it is because of the life they shared I am able to spend time with my family. There is not a price tag that anyone can place on such a valuable gift.

Everyday I get to spend with my husband and my two children I count it a blessing. Having the freedom to pick up and go anytime is really wonderful.

My husband and I were able to leave the country for over a week. We spent our honeymoon over in the Bahamas. During the time I was undergoing hemodialysis, I would not have been able to leave the country. I was always concerned about dialyzing in other units. I couldn't even imagine dialyzing in another country. Thank God it is a new day. Living with a new kidney is like being a new person. In addition to, the kidney I was a newlywed. My children and I had to adjust to living with someone. I was also adjusting to my newfound health. It had been eleven years since I was healthy.

"Another Unexpected Test Of Faith"

As things began to mellow out, than came the real test of our marriage. Six months after saying I do we took a late honeymoon in the Bahamas. We were on a cruise ship, when I began experiencing joint pain. I ignored the pain because I wanted to enjoy our trip. Towards the end of the trip I was in excruciating pain. I went to the doctor immediately after we returned home. The pains became so severe; I began experiencing sharp pains all through my body. The pain became so intense; it was unbearable to live with. The doctor ordered all types of test. Although I underwent numerous tests, the doctor could not find the source of my pain. She began prescribing strong painkillers. I hated taking pain pills. I was taking enough anti rejection medication for the kidney. Adding one more pill to twenty-two pills might not seem like a lot to the doctor but it was too much for me. I felt that the pain pills were not a solution to my problem. The pain pills only pacified the problem. I was tired of feeling drugged up. The pain pills did not even relieve the pain. Over time the pain grew worst. I hurt so badly I did not want to leave the house. I began staying in the house all the time. There were many nights I had to go into emergency to receive pain injections and a muscle relaxer. The injections would not relieve the pain but they would knock me out. It became impossible for me to work.

The pain became so bad I was literally bed ridden. I became so depressed because of becoming totally dependent on

73

my husband. From the time my husband arrived home from work, he was taking complete care of the children and me. He was working eight hours a day, cooking, cleaning and driving the kids to school. Ted and I were both concerned about how we were going to survive on one income. We were left with no other alternatives. It was impossible for me to return back to work. I could not do anything without being in pain. Both of us went into continual prayer and believed the Lord would make a way. I saw so much pain and agony in my husbands face. I thought he was so disappointed in me. He told me it could be him and that no matter what he was my husband and he loved me.

It seemed like my condition grew worse by the second. There were times I would get up and totally loose my balance. I fell down so much I broke three of my ribs on both sides. On top of it all I had suffered a lot of bone damage after the four years of being on hemodialysis. The treatments made my bones very weak. My ribs began to heal very slowly. I can remember telling my husband to leave me. I was in so much pain and felt so bad about myself. I thought it would be better for him to go away. I was not use to anyone taking care of me. Also I did not want to be a burden on anyone. My husband continuously waited on me hand and foot.

With being in so much pain it was unbearable and I prayed for the Lord to take me home. I had to start walking with a cane when I would go out anywhere. I never knew when I was going to loose my balance and fall down. My ribs were already broken and I could not afford another break. I could not turnover in bed or get up without assistance. Being a young thirty-year-old vibrant woman reduced down to a fragile old shell was hard to deal with. If I had to stay in the state I was in, I just literally wanted to die.

After a year of suffering, I found a specialist who correctly diagnosed the source of my pain. The specialist read through my previous doctors diagnosis. He told me that he did not agree with the previous doctors report. I told him the doctor did not give me a diagnosis. This is why I was in his office. He said, *well according to the diagnosis you have bone cancer.* I was shocked my doctor never shared the diagnosis. I told him well I don't agree with the diagnosis either. All I was given was pain pills and suffered for almost a year. I was desperate to try anything after suffering a year with this condition. The doctor told me, *due to the many years of being on hemodialysis my parathyroid became over accelerated. With the parathyroid being over accelerated my bones have become deprived of calcium.* He said, *there was only one way to correct the condition and that would be through a procedure called a Parathyroidectomy. The parathyroid surgery consisted of removing three and a half quarters of my parathyroid.*

He explained to me that everyone is usually born with four parathyroid. Two on each sides of the neck. The surgical procedure would require the doctor slicing open my neck in order to remove them. He said, *"once I had the Parathyroidectomy the pain would completely dissolve. The worst part of the surgery could be a loss of my voice permanently. However the odds were very low that I would."* Weighing the pain I was experiencing made me desperate to try anything.

There were friends and family that suggested I not have the Parathyroidectomy Surgery. Because they knew so many people that lost their voice. All I knew was I lived in so much discomfort and could not go on the way I was. I am glad I followed my heart and had the Parathyroidectomy. Like the doctor said, *"the pain dissolved immediately."* I have not been in any pain since. And I still have my voice. As I am now writing about the pain it is hard to believe I had endured so much. I often think about the marriage vows that say for good or bad, better or worst, in sickness and in health. We thought about the beginning of our marriage, which seemed so bad at times, but it has actually made us much closer. We know our best days are ahead of us now.

Experiencing the bad makes us better able to appreciate all the good in our lives. If we only had the good we would have fallen apart in times we should have remained calm. Now when something comes our way we both say, *this too shall pass.* Even our children have learned trouble don't last always. It is not to say the situation is comfortable, but we don't fall apart because we know where we have placed our trust. There are times throughout the years we have been truly tested but we have come through together. I believe our children through our endurance have the confidence they need to make it through in life.

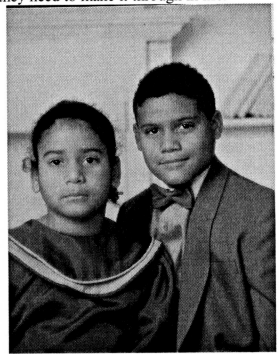

Photograph taken by Hicks Studio 1995
Photo of my two adorable children at the time Daniel was *(eight)* & Patricia was *(seven)*.

Daniel and Patricia both keep me going and always having something to look forward too. They have grown up so fast. I love the two of them so much. They don't really know how hard it was at times to keep pressing forward when I did not have a lot energy. Many times the treatments zapped all of my strength. They both gave me a reason to get up and keep going on. If there is one job I am most proud of I would have to say it has been with these two. Any parent would be proud to have children like them. It doesn't matter how many awards or degrees I have, I'd trade in everything for just my family. We have been through so much together.

However, we have come through it all stronger then ever. We are still a family.

"The Value Of Education"

I've tried to exemplify my educational values through practice. In fact my son and daughter are my first pupils. My two children know that education is one of the most valuable keys to success. They have the same passion and motivation for learning as I do. They are real champions. They live what they are everyday of their lives. I have taught them both that doing a little bit each day over time can go a long ways. *I realized years ago we are who we are before we get to where we're going, not once we arrive.* Our arrival is only a manifestation of what God already had for us. Another one of my great mentors says it all in one of his great words of wisdom.

"Men don't become champions in the ring; they become champions in their routine" -Dr. Mike Murdock

Therefore we are already who we are in the beginning, but as we dig deep we uncover what was already predestined. Both of my children have been on the *Honor Role* since the first grade. They are currently high school students and have maintained an Accumulative 4.0 GPA. They've both been inducted into the National Honor Society. Both of them were Awarded The Who's Who of High School Scholarship incentive, *(The Who's Who of High School is a scholarship worth up to $200,000 towards their educational goals.)* They both were selected into the (ISP) Incentive scholarship Program *(the ISP is a scholarship program where they both will be receiving a full four-year scholarship package from the University Of Michigan upon graduating high school.)* They have so many achievements I have not even began scratched the surface of what they've accomplished.

Another thing I have taught them both, is that applied knowledge is power and to value their education. They exemplify all the qualities that go in conjunction with what they've learned. My children have watched all that I have endured and have discovered there isn't anything they can't accomplish. Through my experience they've learned a person is not limited by an illness, only where they limit themselves. Their teachers ask me how do I keep them so focused and excited about school?

It has been through a lot of steadfast prayers and daily pleading the blood of Jesus over their lives. In addition to getting involved in whatever they're doing at school and other activities. Even during the times I have not felt my best, I had to be there for them. I've made it a point to know who their friends are. I know if we don't discuss things with our children someone else will. What I've learned most through raising children is they learn by example not through lecturing. Children imitate what they see not what they are told.

It is my dream to show another person there is a way out. Through education they will be able to climb heights never imagined before. This is why I have chosen education as my goal. There is always room for improvement and education is one of the paths to steers us towards the direction of developing our best pieces of work. I know for me I have not experienced my best day. I have not drawn my best portrait, and I have not written my best book. Through educating others I play a hand in another life achieving success.

I hope ESRD patients will learn something of value through my experiences. If there is but one thing a patient walks away with I hope they realize *trouble don't last always;* it doesn't matter what you're dealing with, this too shall pass. Knowing that your circumstance is only temporary can be a powerful revelation in itself. Your destiny is locked up in getting tomorrow's desired results. That means every step you take right now gets you one step closer to your desired tomorrow coming to pass.

Through the power and guidance of the Holy Spirit, He has given you a unique ability to strive after the greatness on the inside of you. There is a true champion on the inside waiting to arise and take his rightful place.

Be always willing to make sacrifices to become more then what you are. You have the power "Right Now" to change everything in your life. The enemy will try to tell you this is not for you. You might have even failed in the past but it is a new day. *Therefore, get back up and get back into the race! It is not about how many times we fall down it is how we finish our course.* As long as there is still breath in our bodies we can make it happen.

There are small steps you can start with right now. Once you receive your transplanted organ make a commitment to some daily habits of keeping track of your vitals and weight. These habits should become a natural part of your daily routine.
Start out with these basic habits in the chart below.

Monitor these four *Daily*

VITALS	MEASUREMENT
Take Your Pulse	60-100 beats per minute
Monitor your Blood Pressure (BP)	A normal BP is around 120/70
Take Your Temperature	A normal body temperature is 98.6 Patients should report all temperatures that are 100.5 or higher.
Maintain Your Weight	Patients should be careful not to have too much of an excessive weight gain also obsessive weight loss can be a problem too

Information in Charting Retrieved from The Transplant Patient Partnering Program By Roche Laboratories Inc. 2003 for more information call: 800-893-1995 or visit www.tppp.net

It is not only receiving the transplant that should be a patient's primary focus. Keeping the transplant by remaining healthy should be their ultimate goal. This is how we show a donor we appreciate that gift of life.

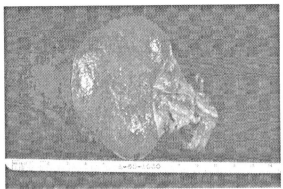

*Photograph of a patient's kidney Afflicted with End Stage Renal Disease of chronic glomerulonephritis. The patient is a 38-year-old man who is presented with the onset of the three signs of uremia; 1. Loss of appetite, 2. Lethargy 3. Increased BUN. The patient has had no previous history of acute glomerulonephritis of Renal1: ESRD Retrieved on April 4, 2004 from:*www.som.tulane.edu/classware/pathology/medical_pathology/McPath/G.

8

Accepting Loss

Surely He shall not be removed forever; the righteous shall be in everlasting remembrance (Psm. 112:6).

Throughout the years I have had to deal with a lot of loss. Even though I've had to move on with my life; losing someone I've loved will always be a part of me. Eventually I've learned I can live with it but I'll never get over it. There are times now, I still think about my mom. She's been dead over eleven years and it almost seems, as though it was just yesterday; she was fussing at me about something. I can even remember my best friend Demetrous, telling me about a lot of the clients that he was working with. Either he was coming up with some brilliant design or putting the finishing touches on another one. He was an awesome artist. If I reminisce a little bit longer, I can remember Nanette getting married and receiving her 2nd kidney transplant operation. But if I blink too long; than painfully I can remember her losing her 2nd kidney transplant. Nanette immediately returned back to hemodialysis for the last time; when I received my 1st kidney transplant. It is hard to believe that such a young vital life is here one day and gone the next. It is still painful for me to talk about her death.

My memory of another patient Vera is a person that always made treatments very interesting for me. She was constantly complaining about how she hated coming to treatments week after week. She would complain and keep track of all the patients that passed on. Vera did not find any point in us all coming to treatments because we were going to eventually die anyways. I think a lot of times Vera liked to depress herself. She never really meant any harm but it was the way she learned how to cope. This is why I've said, *everyone handles dialysis differently.*

As I began digesting a lot of the pain throughout the years; the losses became very devastating to deal with. Most young people my age would think about what they're going to wear to their first date or getting married. I was trying to determine if I'd make it through my next treatment. Dealing with a lot of the adversities along the way has been very devastating for me. Especially since a lot of the young patients passed on were suffering from the same condition I was. Although I had been blessed with a cadaver kidney transplant a lot of my friends did not make it out alive and died waiting. Sure I was grateful I was still alive but the pain of losing a lot of my friends still lives with me. Not being able to talk about what I was dealing with was even more painful. I could no longer call Demetrous, Nanette or Vera. No one else could share my pain. We were there for each other.

Other people that have never suffered with ESRD don't mind being there for you in the beginning but after a while people get tired of you. It is sort of like when I first got ill people seemed to be there for me. After a while most of them began to see it was something ongoing and therefore eventually they seemed to dwindle away. That is why I have learned not to share a lot of my pain. It is okay to go through something. However, people don't like you going through too long. After a while they began to think you should be over things by now.

"The Grievance Process"

Loosing your kidneys can be a very devastating shock. There are five stages of grievance all ESRD patients go through. Every patient goes through and handles each stage very differently. The five stages are *Denial, Anger, Bargaining, Depression,* and *Acceptance.* The stages are much like dealing the process of *death* and *dying.* It sometimes takes a while to get to the final step of acceptance.

I remember dealing with this first stage *Denial* for long time. Denial is the stage where a lot of ESRD patients get stuck at for a very long time sometimes years before starting their treatments. They also deal with denial for a little while after they begin treatments. But usually after going through the treatments they began to realize that it is something they have to do. There are other patients that get stuck at a cross between stages one and two. Either they are in denial about what they are going through in addition to being angry they have to go through it.

Although *Depression* seems to be the third stage in the process, I some how would feel *Bargaining* can some how jump to the first stage. A lot of times ESRD patients try to bargain with God about getting out of what they are going through. Then there are some patients that jump through the first few stages right to depression. They would rather die then be stuck on a machine the rest of their lives. They cannot see themselves as more outside of the dialysis unit. Then there are the patients that make a smooth transition right through to *Acceptance.*

"Praise Him Through It All"

I have learned to give the Lord the praise in advance. It is important to have a relationship with the Lord. Don't just praise Him because of what happens in your life. Praise Him because of who He is. It is easy to say you love someone when they do something wonderful for you. But the Lord is wonderful all the time. He is always doing something good for us even when we don't realize it.

I am sure that you might have heard the phrase don't wait until the battle is over shout now. Shouting after the fact does not prove your faith. It is what we do while you're going through the trial that is a true testament of what you believe. Before I received my transplanted organ I was giving the Lord the praise. Praise is what I do, and worship is who I am. It is not good to only praise when things are going well in your life. Oh no you need a foundation to stand on. A solid foundation is going to sustain you through and through. God is Good all the time. You are still alive no matter what you are living with. I often feel like David when he said,
I will bless the Lord at all times and His praises will continually be in my mouth.

The Lord is good all the time. He is always working out the good on our behalf. There are things the Lord is working out for us we don't even know about. I always pray for the Lord to go out before me and make all the crooked places straight.

By the lifting of my hands and praising Him, I know my blessings will follow. When the praises go up the blessings will come down. I dare you to praise Him. The enemy doesn't like it when you praise the Lord. We possess three of the most powerful weapons on this earth. Praise is one of our most powerful weapons against the enemy. When we are praising the Lord fear can no longer set in. The second most powerful weapon that we possess is prayer. The third most powerful weapon is to speak the word.
Faith cometh by hearing and hearing by the word of God (Rom. 10:17). The more we saturate ourselves in the Word of God; the more we believe.

For a long time I use to think only reading the word was powerful. But my life was completely transcended when I began reading and speaking the word out of my mouth.

Speaking the word unleashes a power that is truly revolutionizing. If you don't see results right away, just keep on reading and speaking the word. Only the word we speak and believe in our hearts become truth to us. If you think about how the devil tried to tempt Jesus. Jesus spoke the word. We have to learn by His example to practice speaking the word. What we continue to read, hear and speak becomes real to us. We have to believe the Lord will deliver us. Before we know it, we are walking in our deliverance.

"Only Speak What You Want To See"

No matter what opposition you're facing don't speak the negative circumstances out of your mouth. (Heb. 11:3) says, *Through faith we understand that the worlds were framed by the word of God, so that things which are seen are not made of things which are seen, which were not made of things which do appear.* The world believes that seeing in the natural is believing. This is quite the contrary for us as believers. Believers know that we must believe before we see it in the natural. We than have to walk, talk and stand until what we want to see comes to pass. It is never a question of if it will happen it is always a matter of when.

There is nothing that you're going through right now in your life the Lord won't bring you out. If He doesn't remove it He will give you what you need to make it through. There is nothing too hard for God. All we have to do is hold on and continue to trust in Him. If it is too hard for man it is just right for God. (Matt. 19:26) says, *But Jesus beheld them and said unto them with men this is impossible, but with God All things are possible.*

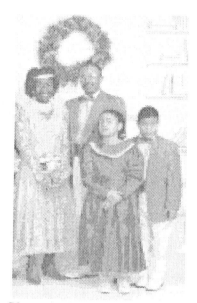

Photographs Hicks Studio 1995
Me (first far left), husband Ted (second left), son Daniel (right) and
daughter Patricia (right center)

9

You Can Make It

I shall live and not die but declare the works of the Lord thy God.
(Psm 66:16)

I am determined no matter what happens in my life, there is
nothing the Lord and I cannot handle. Once you come into
agreement that no matter what you are faced with, you can make it
then you will. As long as you got the God of all creation living on
the inside of you nothing will be able to overtake you? He has
already promised to never leave you nor forsake you. There is
nothing that can move you out of Gods hands.

Paul said in (Rom. 8:35-39), *who shall separate us from the
love of Christ? Shall tribulation, or distress, or persecution, or
famine, or nakedness, or peril, or sword? As it is written, for thy
(Christ) sake we are killed all day long; we are accounted as sheep
for the slaughter. But in all of these things we are more than*

conquers through Him that loved us. Therefore there is nothing that can overcome you.

Paul also lets us know that no matter what we are going through it will never separate us from the love of Christ. He goes on to say in verse 38; *For I am persuaded that neither death, nor life, nor angels, nor things present, nor things to come,*

Obviously Paul thought it was imperative to go on to tell us how deep the love is Christ has been extended to us. In verse 39 Paul continues to say, *Nor height, nor depth, nor any other creature, shall be able to separate us from the love of God, which is in Christ Jesus our Lord.*

I am convinced like Paul there is nothing that can separate me from the love of God, which is in Christ Jesus. If I make my bed in Heaven, He is there or if I make my bed in Hell, He is there too. There is nothing I go through the Lord will not be there to bring me out. You can make it out too!

"Never Swayed By Sight Or Feelings"

No matter what you are faced with, just call on Him. Just think about it, how can ESRD separate you from the love of God? *He cannot lie; He will be with you until the end of the age.* I've had a lot of close calls with death. Many of times it seemed like it was all over but I'm Still here. We don't always have to feel Him to know He is working for us. It is not about a feeling. We cannot trust our feelings. That is why we walk by faith and not by sight. Don't be troubled by what you see. Continue to trust and believe in Him. As long as you continue to believe trust and speak His word; it has to come to pass. It is only a matter of time just keep daily watering the situation with the word of God. He will bring it to pass.

There is only one guarantee in life and that is; His Word cannot lie. I am a living witness of what God can do. There is nothing the Lord won't do for us, *if we are walking up rightly before Him; and we are putting our trust in Him.*

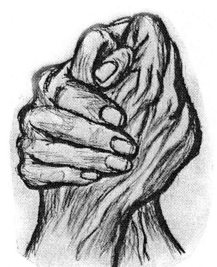

Woman of Strength and Power
Portrait hand drawn by Florence Dyer

10

Moving On In spite of

Behold, the Lord's hand is not shortened, that it cannot save; neither His ear heavy, that it cannot hear (Ish. 59:1).

There is one skill I have learned to master out of all of this. No matter what I'm going through; *I can move on.* I am not saying it doesn't hurt, but I got to get back up and keep on going on. The Lord has delivered me out of toxic relationships, helped me overcome hardship and kept me through devastating losses. He has picked up the broken peaces of my heart and mended them back together again. There were times I didn't think I would live through it all but I did. There were even times I said to myself it was over but it wasn't. I've discovered that I'll rise again in spite of it all.

"Can We Remain Standing"

The one thing that stayed constant throughout, the Lord remained faithful every step of the way. When I speak about the Lord that Healeth it is not only the physical healing. He has healed me emotionally, financially and physically. This doesn't mean that everything has been a bed of roses. In fact it seemed like the more I learned trust in the Lord the more troubles came my way. How would I know Him as a deliverer, if He had never delivered me? How would I know Him as a Healer if He did not heal my body? I would not have known Him as my Provider, if He had never made a way for me. When you ask the Lord for something He has no problem blessing you. The question is do you believe what you're asking Him for?

It is like a book I read once by TD Jakes entitled, *"Can You Stand To Be Blessed?"* Bishop Jakes says, *"the Lord has no problem blessing us, but persecution comes along with the blessing."* This is why he says, *Can You Stand To Be Blessed? Once we are blessed we need to, get ready. Not Everyone is going to be jumping for joy about your blessing. There are some People who will have a problem with your blessing.* He goes on to say, *in fact some people want what you have but they don't want to suffer through what you have to get it.*

Whatever anointing you have on your life, you've paid a great price for it. You will discover the more you become blessed the more people can't stand you. Deep down they probably couldn't stand you from the very beginning. But now the manifestation of the blessings has brought all those deep thoughts right to the surface. I remember when I received the cadaver kidney transplant; it was the happiest day of my life. A lot of the people I fellowshipped with surprised me with their responses. I thought that they would be happy with my deliverance and we would be rejoicing in the Lord together. However the manifestation of my healing created quite the opposite. There seemed to be a lot of envy and strife from people I thought were very close to me. Most of the people had seen me suffering for years.

Their responses were very devastating to me at first. Even one of the young ladies told me that *"if she had to give me a kidney I would die before she would have given me one."* My heart literally dropped to the floor. This is a young lady I allowed to use my car. She had driven me around to my doctor's appointments too. I had never asked anyone for a kidney. Even the Pastor made a public announcement in front of the congregation saying; *yea I love you but you would not have given one of my gizzards.* I have discovered people can be mean, nasty and cruel all wrapped up into one. The bad part about it all is they don't even care. The most frightening thing is most of them are church folk. These are the people I thought would be the most supportive to me.

Although I have constantly had to endure an ongoing battle with ESRD, it has not stopped me from pursuing my dreams. I refuse to allow anything or anyone to determine what or how I can live my life. I have always continued to enjoy whatever I wanted to do. Sure there are days I don't always feel my best but there is always tomorrow. Everyday that my head is above the ground is another day for me to move one step closer to achieving my dreams. Never let anyone or anything tell you what you can have in this life, *if you can see it you be it.* The day I allow ESRD to dictate my life is the day I die. I will always continue to reach for the stars. As long as there is breath in my body I will keep going.

Dialysis has taught me to value every precious moment in life. I have had friends that have died from what I am living with everyday. Living in the midst of death does tend to give ESRD patients a different prospective on life. I realized I'm living on borrowed time. This world is not my home I am just a stranger passing through. I plan to leave this place not carrying anything. *We are known by what we share not for what we bare.* It does not benefit me to keep everything to myself that I know can help someone else. I plan to die empty. I want to help as many people as I can while I am here.

I know I was kept here for a purpose. Maybe it was for you to have a chance to read this book. The Lord is like that. Sometimes He'll have us strategically set up to bless one another. I may have thought *You're The Lord that Healeth...*was birth for renal patients and God may have a totally different plan for someone else. We never know who the Lord will use us to blessing to. He loves each one of us so much and will go to any lengths to come see about us. We also never know whose path our obedience will cross. All I know is I have been compelled to write this book. If I can touch one heart than it will have been well worth it. You don't have to go through anything alone. The Lord wants you healed. Therefore never despise the method of healing the Lord has for you.

"Opening Our Minds To Healing"

We have to always remember that all healing comes from God. No matter what medium the healing comes to us. If you go to the dentist to have an aching tooth pulled the dentist is a medium God used to heal you. If it wasn't a form of healing why didn't you just pray the tooth would fall out on its own? It is not that the Lord could have not supernaturally made the ache dissolve itself.

There are doctors the Lord has gifted to administer healing to us. We reject the Lord when we refuse deliverance. We place limits on what and how we want the Lord to work in our lives. Remember He is able to do more than you or I could ever think or imagine. We are the ones that place Him in a box. It is sort of like we're saying heal me this way, at this certain time and here is how I want it done. We try to give directions to the manufacturer instead of reading the manual. It is also like you telling your car to run without a battery. The car was designed to run with a battery. We don't even have the authority to tell the manufacturer how to make His creation perform. Our lack of knowledge makes us think that we do. In (Hosea 4:6) He says, *that my children are destroyed for lack of knowledge.* We are destroyed by what we don't know.

11
How to Deal With What Happens

I have learned, in whatever state that I am, therewith to be content (Phil. 4:11b KJV)

We have no control over what happens in life. It does not matter how much preventative remedies we take, we cannot control fate. It doesn't matter how good we are, things just happen. Yes, I believe that bad things can happen to good people. It can almost make life seem so unfair. Nonetheless, it is not about how we are as individuals that matters, but how we deal with whatever goes on. When it comes right down to it your personality does not even matter. We have an enemy that does not care about our personality. (John 10:10) says, *the thief comes but to steal to kill and to destroy.* When you have an enemy he does not fight fair. This is not the time to sort out, if you've been knotty or nice. This is a war! You are in a war for your life!

Therefore, roll up your sleeves, take your stance and arm yourself with the word. It is time to get the word into your spirit like never before. Before I got ill, I had read the word occasionally. I was not a big reader but eventually that is all I began to do. Reading became a natural hobby for me. After reading the word regularly, I became strong in my faith. The Lord dealt with me where I was, instead of where I should've been. Through spending time in the word, I began to totally believe every word of God is true.

"Coming Through By Grace"

There's and old hymn my mother use to sing years ago called, *"It's by the Grace of the Lord, I have come a long way."* While she was prancing through the kitchen stirring up a big pot of stew or washing the daily dishes, she'd be singing. I can still see and hear her walking through the kitchen in her old worn black flowery housedress, singing in her old southern voice:

> *It's By The Grace Of The Lord*
> *I have come a long ways.*
> *It's By The Grace Of The Lord*
> *I have come a long ways.*
> *You've been my bread*
> *Lord, when I am hungry*
> *You've been*
> *My company Keeper,*
> *Oh to see that I*
> *Never, never get lonely*
> *I know that it's, by The Grace*
> *Of The Lord*
> *I have come a long ways.*
> *David said, the Lord is my Shepard*
> *That I shall not want*
> *I am a living witness*
> *That He's been my Shepard too*
> *I know that it's, by The Grace*
> *Of The Lord*
> *I have come a long ways.*

When my mom used to sing this song, I really didn't understand the meaning at the time. Now I knew the Lord for myself; I can truly say it was by *the Grace Of the Lord, that I have come a long ways. He has been my company keeper and I have never again been lonely.* Sure I miss my mom, but there is a peace and a joy I have found in the Lord. No matter what comes my way I know by His grace, there is nothing I can't overcome.

The enemy has tried to stop me on every hand, but no matter what I've overcome. I am glad for the foundation both of my parents instilled in me. Although, I was raised in a broken home, throughout my growing up I maintained a strong relationship with both of my parents. They both had a strong belief in God. They always showed my siblings and I, Christ is the only *Way*, the *Truth* and the *Light*. This is why it is important for a parent to do what (Prov. 22:6) instructs us to do and that is to, *Train up a child in the way he should go; and when he is old he shall not depart from it.* We will always come back to what we know. It doesn't matter how long its been, since you've been away. God has always remained faithful. Your still being alive has proven that. God has never left us. We may have left Him but He has always remained faithful. I'm so glad He was waiting for me with open arms. My life was a mess. I've heard so many ministers testify how the Lord turned their mess into a message. I know that to be the truth, because He did it for me too.

I've been asked if, I regret going through dialysis or having the kidney transplant. Honestly, I would say no. Sure I did not like the suffering I've endured. Hemodialysis is not a walk in the park. With the cadaver transplant, I also had some rough times. However, I've come through both of them still standing. I would not be the person I've become today, had I not experienced what I had. The compassion and understanding I have, came through what I've suffered. It is not about how the suffering was caused. It is about how I handled the situation. That is the true test of my faith.

"Adhering To The Warning Signs"

It was now time for me to go through the next chapter in my life. The cadaver kidney function was gradually deteriorating. It was difficult for me to come to terms with this. My pastor had just died months earlier. I had no one to talk to about what was going on. Trying to get through the loss of my pastor was difficult to deal with. As always I found myself consumed with work. This is the way; I've always sorted through adversities.

12
You Can't Run

"It is time to face things head on, running away only prolongs the inevitable." —Florence Dyer

It doesn't matter how I've tried to deny what was going on, the kidney was still failing. I began to discover the clock was ticking and it was time for me to make a decision. The sooner that I chose a form of treatment, the easier it was to get the ball rolling. There is a six-week healing process, for allowing either a graft site or catheter to fully heal. The more that these procedures are put off, the more my life is put at risk. The doctor had already given me three months. Therefore, it was imperative I make doctors appointments and keep them. There were times I had to push myself, to make the appointments. I did not want to talk about what was going on and seeing the doctors only made me think about it more. Because of the loss of function, a lot of times I would forget a lot of dates. This is why it is great to always have someone with you at the appointments. It was as if overnight I was living the whole 1984 nightmare all over again.

The doctors seem to ask a lot of questions about the first transplant. These were questions I wasn't ready for. However, the doctors had to make sure I was physically and emotionally ready to receive a second kidney transplant. It was very devastating for my husband to really accept I had to go back on dialysis. He became very frightened about the possibility of loosing me. His fears made him became very distant and refused to discuss anything about it. He told me he thought if he didn't talk about it; the matter would eventually go away. My son even seemed to become distant too.

"Dealing With It Anyways"

May 2003

Everyone in my home did not want to talk about it. My son became angry and clung to me all the time. He wanted me to attend every activity he was involved in. I was tired of telling him I didn't feel well, even though I didn't. To a seventeen year old, he does not understand mom doesn't feel well. There were even times he would say, *you never feel well anymore.* These words hurt me so badly. He did not know how much emotional pain I was going through. I had to listen to my body or I would pay later.

There were times I would push myself to attend various activities with my children. After attending the events I would be in the bed for days trying to recover. I soon discovered my family has no idea of what I was going through. It seems like they were being very selfish. While on the other hand they have always been the same way. But the disease had begun to interfere with the things I use to enjoy doing with them. To me it seemed like my family was trying to avoid what was going on. Everyone did not want to say anything about it. This was a time I needed them the most. Now that I look back at everything that was going on, it was a big adjustment for them too. It is not that I looked over how hard it was for them; it's just I had a lot on my plate too. No one could really help me talk about what I was experiencing.

How could my family relate? Sure my children had seen me go through hemodialysis when they were younger. But all they knew was that mom had always handled everything. They felt I had been through the first kidney transplant just fine, so what is the big deal with this one? They felt I would go into the hospital for four or five days and come home to recover. It is difficult to discuss my emotions with people that have never undergone a transplant. They will never know what it is like. I don't really want them too.

Making the transition can be a painful process because it can be a very lonely period in your life. There are not a lot of kidney transplant patients available to discuss what is going on with you. You find different books written on how too loose weight, get rich quick schemes, time management, but there are not many books with techniques on how to wait for a kidney transplant. This is a time where you have to just remain in the word and trust the Lord. No one can help you deal with the transition.

Everyone deals with the experience differently. That is why my motto is to *Educate While You Wait.* The more that you learn about what you can expect from your new organ the better you will be able to manage your health care. With my first transplant I did not know as much about what to expect. I only used what knew from other patients plus I read up on the transplant. But after having the transplant there was a lot I did not know. This is why even in my book I have continuously tried to add valuable resources where patients can gather as much free material to learn about what to expect and what is available to assist patients with treatments.

Since I've been through the transplant twice, it has made me become even more aware of protecting my organ in every way that I can. This means finding out everything pertaining to managing my health care.

13
Making the Transition

Now Faith is the substance of things hope for and the evidence of things not seen (Heb. 11:1).

On January 1, 2002 at 2:30 am

I was rushed by ambulance to McLaren Regional Medical Center. I was experiencing difficulty breathing in addition to dizziness and irritability trying to rest. Upon arriving in the emergency room treatment area, the standard lab work was run. Also the oxygen level in my blood was 100%. Every test came back negative which puzzled the doctors; because the symptoms persisted. I urged the doctors to run further test. After running a blood gasket the doctor discovered I needed four pints of blood. This caused for me to stay a few days in the hospital. This was a very difficult times especially since my pastor was also in the hospital fighting for her life. Upon being released from the hospital a few weeks later I found out my cousin was dying from cancer. I attended his funeral on January 23, 2003. It was difficult adjusting to the loss of my cousin. Once I thought things could not have gotten any worse, my pastor died of Leukemia on February 18, 2003. Both of these deaths took me by surprise. Two of the most wonderful people I've ever known gone too soon. In the meantime my health continued to decline. Life is about making transitions. We are always making a transition from one place to another. The success of our transition is based on how swiftly we move into the next place.

On March 30, 2003

I told I had only a few months to live, which was not exactly an easy transition for me to receive. Although I had walked down this path before, I was not ready to do it again. It had been eight years since the last time I was on hemodialysis. I remembered the discipline it took to be a self-care hemodialysis patient. I did not know if I still had the drive in me to endure this process all over again. However, with the possibility of getting a *Related Donor Kidney* this time around gave me a lot of hope. It also gave me even greater concerns I never had before. My siblings were never considered as possible donors when my brother and I were first diagnosised because the doctors were not certain if they would develop the disease. Now it was twenty years later and the odds of them contracting the disease was very slim.

Receiving the 1st cadaver kidney transplant was a much smoother transition on my part. Although the cadaver transplant was a very serious surgery, I had never done it before. My primary responsibly was to receive the kidney when it arrived. When a cadaver kidney arrives there is not enough time to make a lot of preparation before surgery. It all happened so fast and most of the evaluation process has already been completed. There are a few test to make sure there are not any changes. Finally, I just had the option of saying yes or no when it arrived. I realized my decision was a very serious one but I did not have a lot of time to decide.

The 2nd time around became a lot more stressful to me. First of all the transplant coordinator cannot even set up a surgical date until they are certain the donor and the recipient has passed all of the evaluation procedures. This can be a very frustrating process because everything I did or didn't do went against me having the second transplant operation. Even though the process was stressful there were a other things that bothered me more. Not only was I facing a serious surgery, my brother was also facing an even greater challenge. My brother Frank had never had a major surgery before. He could only imagine how serious the surgery was going to be. The doctors informed us both about all of the risk. With my brothers calm demeanor, I don't really think he fully understood how serious the surgery was going to be. I was also bothered by the fact my brother was undergoing such a sacrificial process for me. There is no price tag a person can put on such an enormous gift like this.

The strain on my husband was another matter, which bothered me. He felt helpless that he could not be a donor. Two years prior to me getting ill my husband was stricken with a very debilitating neurological disorder. Because of the neurological disorder he could not be considered as a donor. There are times he undergoes a lot of difficulty with the condition. This was something weighing very heavy on me as well. The enemy has tried in every way to attack our marriage. I know that his plans to destroy have always been through the area of my health. Now he has tried to kill my husband too. The only thing we can do is trust in the Lord. I can identify with Job when he said, *thou He slay me yet will I trust Him.*

I tried my best throughout the entire waiting process to stay focused on other things. I knew if I thought about it too much it would really make the transition a lot harder. I was not new to surgery and I was never concerned about the outcome of the surgery. I knew the Lord was going to keep my brother and me. No matter what we were going through we were coming out victoriously. The Lord had always brought me through. I have always lived my life believing this way for over twenty years and I couldn't think any other way. It was too late for anyone to convince me otherwise.

I will only trust in Him and not lean to my own understanding. The track record I had with the Lord was far too long, to doubt Him now. I have developed a relationship. Trusting in Him is the only way I knew how to get through it all. I learned throughout the years, I couldn't do anything to change the situation anyways. Instead of concerning myself about the outcome I continued to work through my classes and create more designs. Keeping busy has always helped me to move forward. I believe a lot of these adversities in our lives come as distractions to throw us off our course. This is why it is important to never allow what you're experiencing to distract you from your purpose.

This time around is much different than the first. It is now eight years later and I'm married with children. At first my children were nearly babies but they saw me endure it all. Now returning back to dialysis was something new for my husband. It was really a test of our relationship. Couples never know how much their relationship can withstand, until it has been truly tested.

99

Our relationship has gone through many test and trials but we've come out on the other side still standing together. We're vastly discovering each day of our lives; our best day is still ahead of us. Each day of my life I am intrigued by challenge and growth. Going through this process has only strengthened our marriage. What the enemy meant for destruction has only brought us closer together. Now it doesn't matter what he brings our way as Pat Robinson says in his book *"Bring It On."* I am ready for whatever he brings my way. There is nothing the Lord won't bring me through.

"The Loss Of The Cadaver Kidney"

The Nephrologist (Dr. Zaki) kept me on a low dosage of the same transplant medications, while I was undergoing CAPD. He wanted to make sure my system did not have to get use to the anti rejection meds once again. Also the transition of anti rejection meds would make my system better able to handle the higher dosages much easier.

When I had the first kidney transplant; the doctors started me out on a series of anti-rejection medications Including the following: Cyclosporine, Imuran, Minipress and Prednisone. But the doctors discovered I was allergic to the Cyclosporine and Imuran. The meds were not stabilizing my Creatinine.

The Creatinine measures Creatinine levels in the blood and helps to show the kidney is functioning properly. A rise in the Creatinine is an indication the kidney is decreasing in the level of function. Therefore the lower the Creatinine the better the function.

Because of the rise in function the doctors switched me to Neural and Cellcept. My system had a lot of side affects with the combination of the two drugs and I had to be switched to Prograf (Tacrolimus). Because of the increase in my Creatinine level I loss a lot of permanent function that was never fully restored. It took a lot of adjustments until the doctors found medications that stabilized my kidney function. I remained on Prograf, Cellcept, Dilantin, Prednisone, and Minipress (to control my hypertension).

Once the cadaver kidney began to deteriorate the doctors treated me with Epogen injections (three times a week) to help build up my red blood cell count. As the kidney deteriorated further; I was treated with intravenous Iron treatments. I also began experiencing a lot of acid reflux that was treated with Protonix. Large quantities of Calcium were also added to the list of medications to treat the bone damage I had experienced.

Now with the new kidney the doctors have only prescribed the Prograf, Cellcept and Prednisone. They began me on a high dose of each anti rejection med. and have gradually tapered me off as my body began to respond well to the new kidney. The doctors wanted to avoid treating me with High Blood Pressure Medications. So far I have not had to take anything.

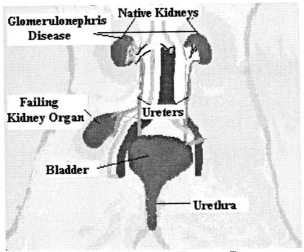

Glomerulonephris Disease

Native Kidneys

Failing Kidney Organ

Ureters

Bladder

Urethra

Photograph drawn by Florence Dyer

14

Another Form of Treatment

For He hath said, I will never leave thee nor forsake thee (Heb. 13:5 b)

When I was told the news about the cadaver kidney transplant failing, it came as a total shock. Although I had always known it was a possibility; knowing and accepting is two different things. However, there was a great deal from my past experiences which helped me deal with the news. I had been through dialysis before and the same God that was with me then will bring me through again. I did not even want to think about going back. In fact I told my husband if I went back to hemodialysis I'd rather die. I refused to even consider hemodialysis. It was okay when I was younger, but I lead a very busy lifestyle and I knew hemodialysis was not for me. I had even worked with CAPD patients before. But as I said with hemodialysis, you never know something until you're going through it.

"Making The Adjustment"

I started CAPD training on May 12, 2003. It took me about three sessions to get the process down pack. Although I knew CAPD was going to be a temporary form of treatment it was important for me to learn everything I could. The more I knew how to manage my own care the better I did with my treatments.

However carrying around the extra fluid took a little getting use to at first. After a while it became a normal way of life for me. Although the treatments took a little bit of adjustment being at home with my immediate family made things much easier. In fact it made it very convenient for me to work on my designs. During my treatments while working on my computer became a normal state of being. Since my work and my classes were both online I knew this would be the best place for me to do my treatments. My family was a lot of help. There were times it was difficult for me to prepare my treatments. It is wonderful to always have a great support system. When you're going through any form of treatment make sure you've surrounded yourself with a great support system. My church family was also a great support system for me. There were times I would get down while waiting for my brothers to be evaluated. Everyone was really an encouragement to me.

It was a blessing that three of my brothers were willing to be tested. This gave me something to look forward too. Being free for eight years made it very difficult to rely on another person. There were so many mixed feelings that were swimming through my head during the evaluation process. No matter what making it a point to not speak about the anxiety was really terrifying. All I knew was that trusting in the Lord was the only way to make it through.

During my wait for the evaluation process to be complete I spent the time as I had before, staying busy. Depending on the type of treatment you've chosen will determine what type of diet that corresponds best with the type of treatment. Because I enjoy eating this is why I chose CAPD. With CAPD I was able to eat more foods in order to keep my strength up. However once having the transplant there were a lot of eating habits I had to control. It is important to exercise and eat healthy as you're waiting and after receiving the transplant. The *Patient Partnering Program* has free pamphlet that gives more extensive details on how to use the 30 % rule.

The rule should be applied to everything that patients eat. Below is a chart that will give transplant patients a brief sample of the 30% rule

DIET	INTAKE
Carbohydrates	40%
Protein	30%-40%
Fat	30%
Calories	30% total percent of calories eaten over several days

Information in Charting Retrieved from The Transplant Patient Partnering Program by Roche Laboratories Inc. 2003 for more information call 800-893-1995 or visit www.tppp.net

The transplant team and dialysis staff can only give patients the facts. The more patients take on an active role in their healthcare the better they will do with any form of treatment. When it all boils right down to it, you're the only one that can make sure you're the best at whatever choices you make. This is why it is important to know what type of diet and activities will keep you functioning at your very best.

According to (James. 2:17) *Even so Faith if it have not works it is dead. Faith* is an action verb, which means it is alive. We do what we believe. At a certain stage in our walk, we are expected to act on our faith. If we believe in health and healing, we are to act accordingly. Too much is given much more is required of us. What was okay with one form of treatment, will not work for another. Just like it is with ever increasing faith. In the beginning believing God is real was okay for that moment in time. But now as you've grown there is a different expectation with each stage in your Christian walk. It is that way with any relationship. In the beginning of a relationship, it was okay to say I love you. After a while there is a different expectation required from you. You are now expected to show your love.

With hemodialysis there were a lot of fluid restrictions placed on me. While on the other hand with CAPD there were hardly any restrictions on fluid. In fact on CAPD I was expected to increase my fluid intake. There is a balancing game required for hemodialysis, CAPD and the transplant.

Each form of treatment is different; just as there is a difference with each transplant. With the cadaver transplant I did not have a lot of fluid retention. However with the related kidney, I have more fluid retention. With the cadaver transplant from the beginning the Creatinine level ranged from 1.9 - 4.0 and throughout the duration of the kidney the levels were up and down. But with the Related Kidney Transplant my Creatinine Levels have remained between 0.9 – 1.0. Also there are fewer medications I'm taking with the *Related Kidney Transplant*. This is why we cannot get caught up in one way of handling a situation. With my second transplant it is like starting all over again. You never know what you've had until you loose it. May times we take for granted being able to urinate. It seems like an automatic function which requires no thinking. However, it is one of the most important functions in our every day existence. The entire process happens without warning. All we are left with is making a choice to deal with it. Sometimes with new experiences we have to throw out everything that we know. Sometimes we can get too complacent with one way of thinking. I could not rely on what I knew about hemodialysis before. I had be open to new experiences and willing to live life one day at a time.

15
The 2nd Time Around

"God is a God of Second Chances." "The 2nd time can be better than the 1st."

My first rejection episode with the cadaver kidney transplant was not a pleasant experience for me. There were times I even thought about never considering another kidney transplant. After my last rejection episode, I lost a lot of kidney function. My creatine level became stabilized at a 4.5, which was very high. I was never able to regain back the function that was lost. Even though my creatine level was high the kidney was still functioning and I remained off of dialysis. The doctors informed me that I was blessed, to still have the function I had left. Most other patients once they have had one rejection episode the kidney usually went out. It was truly a blessing to have survived as many rejection episodes without the kidney going completely out. However, because of the loss of kidney function my red blood cells were no longer able to reproduce on their own. In order to reproduce these blood cells I had to self-administer Procrit (Epogen) injections. The injections were given three days a week. The Epogen injections helped to reproduce red blood cells. The increase of red blood cells gives the body more energy.

The doctors did everything they could to monitor and maintain the remaining function. The most important thing was not being on dialysis for the eight years. I considered myself blessed for being off of dialysis. But I did not want to think about another kidney transplant. My doctor discussed the possibility of considering another operation at some point. While I was very adamant about not discussing it, until it was time for me to cross that bridge.

My husband told me although I had difficulties with the first transplant, maybe the second one would not be the same. He said if I had never took the chance, I would never know if another one would function without any problems. He reminded me *"God is a God of Second Chances."*

"The 2nd time can be better than the 1st"

Well my hubby was right. From the very start this one was totally different. First of all, I had a lot more responsibility of waiting to see if my brothers were compatible donors. Secondly, unlike the first transplant the doctors had a lot more information. The advancements in the surgical procedures and medications had improved greatly. Finally, before my siblings were not considered to be compatible donors. Now they were being considered. During the earlier years the doctors were uncertain, if they would come down with the kidney disease. It had been over twenty years since my brother and I were diagnosed. Today the doctors are more knowledgeable about the disease. Therefore, the doctors were more confident our other siblings were out of the woods.

"Asking Family For A Kidney"

When I went to be evaluated for the 2nd transplant I felt like a complete failure. I was angry that the first one failed. I did not want to even think about starting over. The first year of hoping the transplant didn't reject was very frightening. I was getting nauseated just thinking about the possibility of going through, the process all over again. During the evaluation process the doctors suggested I get all of my siblings tested. I told the doctors I would rather be on the waiting list. The doctors felt I was fortunate the first time around, to receive a kidney so soon. But the wait could be 3-7 years and I could die waiting. The doctors further reminded me about a lot of bone damage I suffered while undergoing hemodialysis. They were concerned about me sustaining more damage.

I decided to ask three of my brothers about being tested. Much to my surprise they all agreed to have the testing done. The tissue testing was a three-week process. During the process my youngest brother changed his mind. He was scared. It was very understandable. However, I could not focus on that right now. Once the results came in about my other two brothers, we were all excited about the news. Both of my brothers were a perfect match. Now it was time for my brothers to decide which one would continue the evaluation process. They decided among themselves our older brother Frank would complete the workup first. If he was not completely compatible my younger brother would do it.

There is a very extensive workup for the recipient and the donor. With the cadaver transplant, I had the option of accepting the kidney or turning it down. This time I had to wait until the evaluation was complete. The workup would show if my brother was completely healthy. This was a totally different area for my family and me. Also my brother had his immediate family to consider too. I was torn with the fact of needing a kidney, my brother's life and our family. If I didn't have the kidney from my brother, it might be years before another one came available. There was a possibility I could die waiting. I felt as though my brother was placed in the position of doing it in order for me to get better. Also I know he probably thought about what the family would say, if he chickened out. I had made peace with myself. If Frank wanted to back out I would understand. Sometimes I thought about never speaking to him again; which would be very hard to do. I love my brother and I could not be that selfish. I had to understand this was a very difficult sacrifice. He never backed down once.

I did not realize the next five months were going to be a real test of my faith. I thought that I knew each one of my brothers. Situations like this bring out the best or the worst in families. Sometimes when you think you know your siblings you discover you really don't. The sibling I thought would be the first one to complete the evaluation process, was not the one that wanted to do it. The other sibling I thought would not go through with it; stuck the entire process out with me. I was amazed to discover the courageousness my older brother Frank possessed. He was there beside me every step of the way. No matter what the doctors informed him about the procedure, he made every appointment. He did not waver in any way.

"Recovering From Surgery"

The doctors were amazed at how fast we both recuperated. My brother was in a lot of pain for the first couple of weeks. I found his pain harder for me to deal with. I felt guilty he was suffering because of me. Over time the pain began to completely dissolve. After going through our follow-up visits, we were both given a clean bill of health. In fact we were both back at church a couple weeks later. My bother was able to return back to work after six weeks. The more I saw him returning back to a normal life the better I felt. These emotions are very normal when you have a living donor.

It doesn't matter if they are related to you or not. Their well-being becomes your number one concern. This was one of the reasons I was always concerned about asking any of my siblings for a kidney. You might be a person wondering how to go about asking a family member for their kidney. It doesn't matter how close you are, it is not an easy thing to ask anybody. This is a part of this person's body. When I asked my siblings I did not know how they would respond and I did not want to ask either. All I knew was that I wanted to live and understood what dialysis was like. For eight years I had grown accustom to the freedom of being off of dialysis.

The only thing I can suggest is that you ask. When you do, be willing to accept and respect their answer. You will be surprised that some of your siblings may not respond the way you think.

It doesn't matter what the enemy brings on, I know the Lord will see me through. I have gotten to the point that I have been through the fire and I have been through the flood. I've decided if I go into the furnace, I know the Lord is yet able. Even if I don't come out, I know it is not because the Lord wasn't able to bring me out. I just believe the Lord will deliver me out of anything. He will do the same for you. All you have to do is trust Him. If you are trusting the Lord for deliverance in any situation don't give up. You hold on, keep speaking and proclaiming your deliverance.

There are going to be times, it might seem like it won't happen. I am here to tell you it will. All you have to do is trust and believe. It will come just for you, with your name on it. When God has a miracle with your name on it, no one else can receive it. When someone else gets blessed with a healing miracle don't get envious. You should be even more encouraged your healing is on the way.

(Isaiah 53:5 KJV) tells us: *But He (Jesus) was wounded for our transgressions, He was bruised for our iniquities: the chastisement of our peace was upon Him; and with His stripes we are healed.*

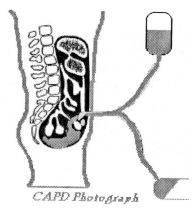

CAPD Photograph

16

Facing Dialysis Again

For the thing, which I greatly feared, is come upon me, and that which I was afraid of is come unto me (Job 3:25 KJV).

I can definitely relate with Job's catastrophe. When the cadaver kidney transplant failed, it was what I feared most. Simply put, *I dreaded the thought of ever returning back to hemodialysis.* Sure I had managed the treatments well. However, I had hoped that stage of my life was over. Even though, I had a few bad experiences with the transplant it was still better than hemodialysis. I did not want to think about being confined to another dialysis machine three days a week. Although, I was able to do pursue my dreams, hemodialysis took a lot of self-discipline. Throughout my treatments, I experienced a lot of infiltration with my fistula and graft sites. It was to the point I barely had an arm left to administer treatments. I didn't even want to consider my legs. These thoughts began racing through my mind.

Some patients have artificial veins in their legs and manage quite well. In that case, there are different strokes for different folks. It was not so much of a vanity issue with me. It was that I had conquered this demon once and now it was back again. Just the thought of starting all over again, is something I did not want to do. I was so angry with myself. I did not want to consider anything. I knew it was not right for me to behave this way. But I had to let my frustration out. What I was facing was unavoidable. This is something I knew all too well. The sooner I began the process of heading in the direction of acceptance the easier it would be for me to overcome. The longer I refused to deal with it, the harder I was making it for myself.

For me to face that the cadaver-transplanted organ failed, was very difficult to accept. To say failure meant to me that I had failed. The doctors tried to reassure me I had done well. They were impressed I'd endured a lot of the various complications with the 1st transplant. To go eight years was more than average for cadaver organ. They said, *"to even endure with the loss of function was even quite and accomplishment."* Although I wanted to beat myself up about it, there was still a decision to be made. What disappointed me most is that I did not have a lot of time to make it. The doctor had given me three months to live.

I began to stay in the house a lot and did not want to really see anyone. My husband was not feeling well and was forced into an early retirement because of his condition. This was one of the most devastating moments in our lives so we thought. We were praying and believing God for deliverance. There were even times neither one of us were able to drive. Our son had just turned seventeen. He had just begun to drive. There was a time I could not see myself allowing him to drive us around, but he did. It seems like he had just gotten his permit during the time all this was going on. I began to discover that starting treatments was going to be a lot different this time around.

"Sharing With Extended Family & Friends"

Telling other members of my extended family was very hard. My aunt was very insensitive about the whole ordeal. She said, *"what is the big deal you've done dialysis before?"* She went on to say, *"you should have known the kidney wouldn't last forever; didn't the doctors tell you this?"* Every word she said was like a dagger in my heart. Tough love is not what I need right now. The doctors never told me how long a cadaver kidney would last. My aunt did not know or realize how bad I was hurting. She had even more great advice on the type of treatment I should receive. She thought I had managed well on hemodialysis. She had no idea of everything I had been through. She has never went to one treatment or checked to see how well I had managed. Reactions like this use to bother me when I was younger. Now I have undergone so much and have chosen to ignore ignorance.

Although, I love my aunt she doesn't understand. I pray to God she never has to experience anything like what I've gone through. People that have never walked in your shoes have no idea about what you go through. *They don't know how much of a blessing it is you're alive to even consider another form of treatment.* I pray the Lord enlightens my aunt and illuminates her heart.

Not everyone is going to be supportive about your choices. That is why there are choices you are going to make regarding your health care, you can't share with everyone. After making all of these negative statements, my aunt was angry I did not include her in every detail of what was going on with me. I was going through another difficult time in my life and could not afford to hear anymore-negative reports. I am sure you may know others like my aunt who always likes to update you on patients that have experienced terrible outcomes. You don't need any negativity with what you're getting ready to go through. For instance, back in 1997 when I was getting ready to have a Parathyroid Surgery my aunt had a dozen bad reports from people she'd run into about why I was making a bad choice in having the surgery. I am sure that you might have been going through something where others have said, *such and such had that same surgery and this and that happened to them after words.* Never mind the fact I was in the most excruciating pain everyday of my life.

All I knew was I could not go on hurting the way I was. I needed some form of divine medical intervention. I did not want to undergo another surgery but I could not stay in the pain that I was in any longer. It was another one of those great decisions that I made. Immediately after the removal of three and a half of my parathyroid the pain totally dissolved. To this very day it is as if I had never suffered the pain at all. After hearing so much negative advice from people, I've just learned to find out what the Lord is saying about the situation.

It is best to pray for Godly friends to come into your life. A lot of them help you vent your frustrations. Ask for friends that won't judge your choices and will be a shoulder to lean on in the rough times. The only thing with having a friend like this, you need to learn to be a friend too. In order to have friends, we have to be there for them too. I have family and so called friends that have reacted negatively to my condition. But I've also been blessed with positive Godly friends too. They've stuck with me through everything I've been through. That is why I can speak from both ends of the spectrum. A real friend does not have to agree with every choice you make. You don't have to always agree with them either. But you both have learned to respect one another in whatever choices that either of you make. The one thing you'll discover most when you're going through is, who your true friends are. The Lord will unveil the people that are not for you. He will replace them with more supportive friends. Even though He blesses you with Godly friends you cannot lean on them for everything.

Going through dialysis the second time around, was much different for me. First of all, I've grown to know the Lord in a better way. Secondly, when I was undergoing hemodialysis I was getting acquainted Him. Finally, not only do I know Him I'm getting to know Him in a deeper way. Having endured the ordeals in the past has increased my faith. It is true when they say what doesn't kill you only makes you stronger. But what I can add to the philosophy is that the strength I've gained is in Him. Tests come to make our faith stronger in Him and the power of His might. I thank the Lord my strength is not in myself.

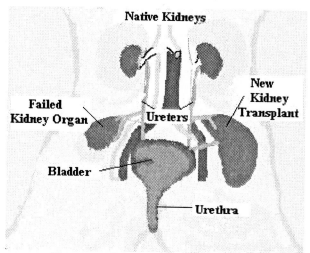

Photograph drawn by Florence Dyer

17

Starting Another Form Of Treatment

Many are the afflictions of the righteous: but the Lord delivereth
him out of them all (Psm. 34:19).

This time around I chose (CAPD) Continuous Ambulatory Peritoneal Dialysis. Having lived through so much I was no longer the little frightened nineteen year old just being informed about having a kidney disease. Also I was no longer the person that went into the hemodialysis unit back in 1991. Throughout the years I had learned a few things that developed me into the person I've become. Based on my knowledge I felt CAPD gave me an entirely new prospective on life. There were things CAPD offered me now; hemodialysis would constrict me from doing. When I was on hemodialysis years ago, I did not know what to expect. All I knew about hemodialysis were from the conversations I had with my younger brother. Also being a self-care patient and working as a Medical Assistant, I had a chance to learn about CAPD and hemodialysis treatments. At this time in my life choosing CAPD was more suitable to my lifestyle. Another reason for my choice was because the hemodialysis nurses had infiltrated my fistulas and a couple grafts while undergoing treatments. The grafts seemed to be a big problem for me.

Years ago a Nephrologist had suggested CAPD to me. I refused CAPD treatments because I did not feel CAPD suited my needs at that time in my life. I chose hemodialysis instead because my children were very young and very active. Having two active toddlers at home was not a great atmosphere to undergo CAPD treatments. My son demanded a lot of my attention and he was very inquisitive. CAPD treatments require patients stay in a very sterile environment. In addition to making exchanges every four to six hours a day (seven days a week). It would not have been the best form of treatment with two small children that were into everything, every minute of the day.

"A New Day And Time"

Now my children are sixteen and seventeen this time around. In addition to them being teenagers I am also married. Unlike the first time I was a single parent balancing everything alone. It is very encouraging to know I have a lot of help as well as a great support system. Most importantly the CAPD exchanges, fit better into my busy lifestyle.

It was readily apparent at this stage hemodialysis was not going to be the right treatment for me. I am more informed and able to make choices that are more conducive to my needs. It is great to know what you don't want in your life as opposed to what you can handle. It would be difficult for me to fit in the hemodialysis treatments in at this stage of the game. There are two drawback I discovered with choosing CAPD. First of all, the exchanges are four times a day, seven days a week. I fully understood the process going into CAPD. Secondly, CAPD requires a lot more self-discipline because it is done daily. In spite of the drawbacks, with each form of treatment there are expectations.

"Tolerance" is one sure thing I learned as a hemodialysis patient, CAPD patient and a kidney transplant patient. No one can

tell me what I can and cannot stand. There is no one is going to be taking the treatments for me. I have real concerns about people when they think they know what is best for my choice in health care. You're the one that has to sit in the chair. Unless another person sits in your place they cannot speak on what is best for you. It is great to discuss your choices but let no one make the choice for your life. This is your life no one else's.

FORM TREATMENT	ADVANTAGES	DISADVANTAGES
Hemodialysis	Three days a week (12-15 hours weekly) Instead of daily like CAPD Patients feel really good when they follow a proper renal diet	Has to be done in a unit or can be done at home with a committed partner Patient is more restricted on various foods has to follow a Renal diet (the patient has to avoid salt, sugar, water, and etc.) Treatments are harder on the patient's body then most other forms of treatments. (Patients suffer more bone damage the longer they undergo treatments) Patients who undergo treatments have to arrange schedules around treatments
CAPD Continuous Ambulatory Peritoneal Dialysis	CAPD Exchanges can be done almost anywhere as long as the atmosphere is	Exchanges has to be done 4-6 times daily Have to have dialysate solution left in at all times.

	sterile. Patient can schedule their exchanges around various activities Patient is not restricted from eating a variety of foods (patients feel really good when they are eating well)	Patients will have bloatedness at all times. Some patients are affected more than others (Patients suffer similar damages as hemodialysis but at a slower pace)

Each form of treatment has its *advantages* and *disadvantages*. We have to weigh what is going to be the most accommodating method for us. I'm not saying which method is going to be the most convenient. None of them will ever be convenient. Whenever we have to do something, convenience goes out the window. There are occasions where patients are not able to choose certain forms of treatments. In either case a patient should always discuss the options that are available before making a choice. There are some patients I have come across who were never told about all of the options available to them. After reading this book hopefully that will no longer be the case. I have purposely taken out the time to lay all the cards on the table for patients to know what is available for them. Never let anyone tell you what will work best for your situation. Neither my husband nor my children were going to be enduring this process. I am glad they never tried to impose their views on what they would do in my situation.

When it comes to a decision about any form of treatment that is going to effect the rest of your life, no one can make that decision for you. It was also great to have the support of my siblings. There were a lot of family functions I had to miss during the treatments and after the transplant surgery. Every year I usually attend our family reunion in Chicago. This year I wasn't up to traveling. I'm sure everyone understood but it did not replace my pain of not being there. It is great memories will last forever. If it's the Lord's will, I am sure I'll make the next family reunion.

I thank the Lord for each one of my siblings being a part of my life. I have learned so much from each one of you. I love all of you so much. I am grateful for your love and support.

Dorothy I thank you for always being a listening ear and being there for me every time I've needed you. You have been a true big sister.

Frank thank you for your kidney which keeps me up all night. I always think of you every time I have to go. I'm sure that makes you smile.

Floyd thanks for your wonderful jokes. I am sure my book will find its way in some of your comedy material.

Fred you are my serious brother. I love you and regardless of how tall you are, you'll always my little brother. It is in print now so you can't erase it. You're taller but I am always going to be older. Stay strong, I love you.

Baton I love you with all my heart and thank you for always *"Keeping It Real brother."*

Lakeshia I love you and I am very proud you graduated from the Paralegal Program. I am sorry I was unable to be there for you. But you know I was there in spirit.

Felexis I wasn't able to make it to your wedding but I want you to know I love you and happy belated congratulations. I was unable to travel at that time but look forward to saying congratulations in person soon.

Benson I want you to know I love you and want you to grab hold of what the Lord has available for you in life.

18
Ain't No Grave

If I wait, the grave is mine house; I have made my bed in the darkness (Job 17:13 KJV)

There are a lot of things that happened along the way I did not expect. I never thought the cadaver kidney would fail. Nor would I've thought I would have one of my sibling's kidney. From the time of being diagnosised with a kidney disease there has been so much that has taken place. In spite of all I've been through; I still have joy. There is always a song in my heart. I come from a family of gospel singers. A lot of times when I am going through various transitions in my life there is a song that rings so true to my heart entitled *Ain't No Grave*. My father recorded this song over thirty years ago. Also I lead the song with my brothers at my mother's funeral. This song was so fitting for my mom's character. *Ain't No Grave* is a song that gives me so much inspiration and hope. Throughout the verses in the song I think about how blessed my mom is to be resting from all the trials and tribulations of this evil world.

There will come a day when Gabriel's Trumpet will sound. The bible says, *"the dead and Christ shall rise first. Those of us that are saved who have remained will be caught up to meet Him (Jesus) in the air."* The words of an old song, *"Ain't No Grave"* give me so much consolation. That is why when I think about death I know it is not final. There *Ain't No Grave* can hold my body down. The song goes something like this:

Ain't No Grave
Ain't No Grave my Lord
Hold my body down
Lord (do, do, do)

Say it Ain't No Grave
Ain't No Grave my Lord

Hold my body down yea
When the first trumpet sounds
I 'm gonna rise up, yea from the ground
I said it Ain't No Grave,
Ain't No Grave my Lord
(do, do, do)

I remember many years ago
When we would go to church
On Sunday morning
Mother use to gather all us children
The Preacher ask us to bow
our heads in prayer
I remember there was an old lady
She would stand up and testify
She would let us know just why

She said, Father I love you
And I believe it, when I die
There ain't no Grave,
Ain't no Grave My lord
Hold my body down
Lord (do, do, do)

There Ain't no Grave,
Ain't no Grave My lord
Hold my body down
When the first Trumpet sounds
I'm gonna rise up from the ground

-*original Author unknown. Revisions have been made to accommodate personal circumstances.*

    I believe like the lyrics in the song, there *"Ain't No Grave that can hold my body down."* I am determined to continue a relentless fight until the end. I received my 2nd kidney transplant operation on October 30, 2003. I feel fantastic and look forward to a long life of good health. This has been a long road but the Lord has certainly kept me and is still keeping me. Although I have endured a great deal I would not trade what I have gone through for anything in the world. Throughout the various adversities I found the Lord. In 1984 I discovered the Lord and He was worth far more than anything that can ever be said about my life.

"My View Of Dialysis"

I view dialysis like sitting in a room with a door closed. The Lord is saying turn the knob and *Open The Door*. He has healing available to you right now. Just turn the knob and open the door. We have to make the first move. He is so wonderful that he will never supersede our will. He loves us so much that he designed all of us to be free will agents. I believe that he hurts when we are suffering especially when he has healing within our reach and we won't receive it.

I believe God hears and answers our prayer. We are the ones who choose to reject His method of healing. Fear as I said before, is one of the most stubborn enemies to ESRD patients. God is constantly sending the doctors around to say there is healing available for you right now. Every time He is trying to send the message to turn the knob and open the door fear causes us to choose to continue sitting in the chair. We continue to look for another form of healing to come. It is not to say that there is not any other form of healing for us. Oh I believe divine healing can come with or without surgery. I sat on dialysis for over three years turning away every doctor that came my way. I did not know it was because of my ignorance in the area of healing I was suffering unnecessarily. The moment I began to move in the direction of my healing my kidney was soon released. It was like almost instantly the Lord sent me confirmation.

"Some Unexpected Surprises"

I thought after the 1st kidney transplant failed my life was finished. Little did I know it was just another opportunity for the Lord to show Himself strong in my life again. At the time I was going through, I could not see any good in what was going on. But it was through the loss of the cadaver kidney my brother was able to be a blessing to me. It was an opportunity for my brother to also experience the goodness of the Lord. Through his giving our family bond become even stronger. We are able to show the world there are African American families that truly love one another and are willing to sacrifice their lives for family. It is not our hope to be a minority in organ donation *but a beacon for others to come forth.*

There is always good in whatever happens. We don't always see the good in the situation right away. Sometimes we are very uncomfortable through the whole ordeal. But if we wait on the Lord, He has promised to renew our strength. If we continue to hold on; we will mount up like the wings of an eagle. I am proclaiming what (Haggai 2:9) says about, *The Glory of this latter house shall be greater than of the former, saith the Lord of Host: and in this place will I give peace, saith the Lord of Host.*

There is such a peace I have in my spirit right now. No I don't always know how things are going to end up but through it all I have discovered no matter what comes my way; *the Lord has it all in control!!!!!!*

God Is Faithful To His Word

On October 10, 2005 I started feeling extremely tired. The symptoms were a lot similar to what I had experienced when my Hemoglobin dropped (in January of 2003). It was as if I was back on the same roller coaster all over again. In addition to feeling tired my appetite had decreased tremendously. Since I've been on this journey there is not much I ignore or take for granted. Therefore I decided to go straight away to have my lab work done. Labs for transplant patients are always sent to the doctor labeled STAT. STAT is a term, which means IMMEDIATE. October 11 the very next day, I went into my doctor's office for a routine scheduled appointment. The doctor had a copy of my lab results. The results revealed that my Creatine was 5.8 with my Hemoglobin at 6.3. My doctor immediately admitted me into Hurley Medical Center. The doctor ordered a biopsy, CBC, Blood Transfusions, High dosages of Sodium Medrol (which is a steroid to treat anti rejection) and a battery of other test. The Dr. was alarmed about the huge blood loss as well as the continual rise in my Creatine Level. The symptoms gave the indication that the 2nd kidney was failing. I did not care what the report was saying I knew God has the last word. I know the Lord does not do anything half way; therefore this was another test of my faith. I had sat in this position too many times. The enemy on the other end was whispering the words I knew all too well; here it goes again, *You are going back to dialysis.* The devil is a liar and a deceiver too. Sure the report was indicating that but I refused to listen. There was no way I was going to let this kidney go. My brother had shed his blood and nearly sacrificed his life to give me this kidney. There was no way I was going to hand this kidney over without a fight. I began to pray and remind the Lord that He said in His Word by His strips I am healed. I did not care what the report was indicating all I knew was what God had done for me. Therefore I am going to stand on His Word.

Once the doctors came into the room to give me the news, I had fully prepared myself for it. The doctor said, I had developed either Acute or Chronic Rejection. If it was Acute Rejection there might be a window of opportunity to reverse the affects. However, if it was Chronic Rejection there was no since in fighting for the kidney. The results of the biopsy would determine how aggressively the doctors would proceed in treating the results. As I waited for the results there was another doctor I knew who has never let me down. I called upon Him in the midnight hour. Before the break of day there was that peace in my spirit that everything was going to be alright. When the doctor came into the room he said, it was Acute Rejection and it could be treated.

However, the result revealed something very unusual. I had developed a rare condition called *Hemolytic Uremic Syndrome. I was puzzled by the news. The doctor told me, he was somewhat familiar with the condition. It is not something that has been seen very often in fact there were only about 30 transplant patients who had developed the condition.* The condition usually was a result of taking Prograf or a viral infection. He also told me *Thrombotic Micro Angopathy* is another name for the condition. *Thrombotic Micro Angopathy is a condition causing small capillaries and arteries to be plugged up with small clots (what was so unique about the condition was the small clots were specifically compounded to the new kidney).* Taking Prograf over an extend period of time was causing the condition. Therefore he was going to be stopping the Prograf ASAP. I was on Prograf with the 1st kidney and now with this one too. This began to make me think back about losing the cadaver kidney. Although it was too late to save the 1st one I could not help thinking about how the loss could have been prevented. It would have been great to discover this information with the first transplant.

I realize that doctors learn as they go too. My kidney function was being sustained with the Prograf and they saw know reason to change. If something is not broke we don't usually fix it. My brother is also using Prograf and may not experience the same results. However, I still made it a point to inform him about what happened to me. I thought this information is important other transplant patients too. Not all patients experience the same effects from Prograf. My doctor informed me that there have been 30 cases found. This discovery was through the University of Michigan. Over time my body had began to develop antibodies against the Prograf. Instead of the Prograf working to sustain the kidney function it began working against the kidney. The doctor immediately switched me from Prograf to Rapamune. Rapamune is *an anti rejection medication that has been on the market for about five years.* With the immediate switch to Rapamune in addition to Plasmapheresis treatments the doctors where hopeful that my levels would return to normal. The doctor told me that the process generally takes a few weeks to see results. The Plasmapheresis treatments were administered every other day. Altogether I had a total of twelve Plasmapheresis treatments.

During the first Plasmapheresis treatment I became very ill because my calcium level was too low. The following five treatments afterwards went very good. There was some irritating itching I experienced during my seventh treatment. According to the pheresis nurse these side effects are quite common. I was given Benydril to combat the irritating itchiness. The Benydril was also given to help me relax. No matter what I experienced the pheresis nurse was constantly on top of everything. The pheresis nurses addressed all of my concerns this helped me to feel more comfortable. Throughout every treatment the one side effect that remained consistent, *was that I felt extremely cold.* This is a side effect every patient experienced. There are ways to help patients endure the cold. The nurses were very good with providing me with plenty of blankets. Through most of the Plasmapheresis treatments, I was covered from head to toe.

Plasmapheresis is a machine similar to a Hemodialysis machine. Although the machines are similar Plasmapheresis does not serve the same function. Unlike a Hemodialysis machine the Plasmapheresis machine does not cleanse the blood. The Plasmapheresis machine removes all of the patient's plasma and exchanges with new fresh frozen plasma; donated by healthy living donors. Exchanging the patient's plasma for fresh plasma allows the infected elevated antibodies built up to fight against the kidney function to be removed during the exchange process. The patient is given new healthy antibodies through the new plasma exchange, which allow the kidney to function in the way that it should. This usually helps the function return back to normal.

I feel like I've been blessed beyond measure to be given an opportunity to afford to have these treatments done. Through the Plasmapheresis treatments and switching to the Rapamune Anti Rejection Medications my kidney function has returned back to normal. I wanted to include this information for other patient who might be feeling the same way. My body told me something was wrong and I listened. Listening to your body does not shake your faith in God. God placed doctors here to assist in administering healing to the sick. The doctor does know everything. But any knowledge that the doctor has acquired came from the Lord. I am glad that the Lord has placed God-fearing doctors in my path. My doctor is a man of faith. Even when he has given me a report he has always told me to be in prayer. This is something I respect about his practice. I am going to continue to take one day at a time. As I learn more on this journey it is my hope to assist other ESRD patients in getting the best quality health care available.

I realize long ago that it is not all about me. Throughout my battles God has shown me I am here to help others. It is not through my suffering but in the process of my trials, I am able to be a blessing to others. Many times I've felt throughout my experience as though I was an experiment. However, once the procedure worked then the Lord has shown me how I can help other patients. Sure I wish I didn't have to endure the pain and suffering but it has worked out for the good. It is not about what happens but how we deal with what happens. Either we are going to use it for the good or allow it to keep us down. Either way we have a choice in the way we allow the experience to effect our lives. I'm sure you've learned through reading You're the Lord that Healeth...not to let anything hold you down. As long as God is before you, what is there in this world that can hold you down but you. God is faithful to His Word. *To God Be the Glory Who Always Causes Us To Triumph In Christ Jesus!!!!!!!!!!*

Below is what God wants for you and me:

(3 John 2) *Beloved, I wish above all things that thou mayest prosper and be in health, even as thy soul prospereth.*

SPECIFIC   MONITOR   CHART   FOR   KIDNEY   TEST
RESULTS

MEASURES	INCREASE	DECREASE
Bicarbonate Acid base balance of blood as controlled by the kidney	A long disorder Taking too many antacids	A sign of diabetes Kidney failure
Urinalysis White blood cells, red blood cells, bacteria and protein levels in the urine	Kidney disease Urinary track infection Poorly controlled diabetes	(N/A)
Protein in Urine Normally protein is not present in urine. Quantity of protein may be measured over a 24-hour period	A kidney disorder A complication of diabetes	(N/A)
Calcium Needed for blood clotting building bones, and also the muscles heart and nerve function	Too much calcium intake Bone disorder Problem with parathyroid or thyroid	Inflammation of pancreas Kidney failure Too little vitamin D Too much water in the body
BUN Blood urea nitrogen Waste product of protein brokendown that is removed from the blood by the kidney's	Kidney is not functioning properly Diet high in protein Dehydration	Liver disease Too much water in the body

MEASURES		INCREASE	DECREASE
Uric Acid	A waste product of energy production found in the urine and the blood	Gout Liver disease or ulcerative colitis	(N/A)
Triglycerides	Fat like cholesterol helps determine the risk of coronary artery disease	Poorly controlled diabetes High blood pressure Risk of coronary artery disease	Malnutrition Overactive thyroid
Cholesterol	Fat like material that helps to make hormones and build cell walls	Narrowing or blockage of blood vessels Side affect from anti -rejection	(N/A)
Creatinine	Measuring Creatinine in the blood helps to show the kidney is working properly	Dehydration Side affect from anti -rejection meds Kidney disease	(N/A)
Sodium	Balance between electrolytes and water in the body	Excessive sodium in diet Not enough water	Chronic kidney disease Inadequate sodium intake
White Blood Count (WBC)	White blood count fight off infection	Infection Inflammation Tissue destruction	Too few infections fighting cells to protect the body taking meds like anti rejection, diuretics or antibiotics

2002 Chart by Roche Laboratories Inc. For more information about Partnering Program visit www.tpp.net Or call 800-893-1995 for more {free} in home library of transplant material.

10 Tips for Traveling With Anti-Rejection Medications

1. Always carry extra medication with you in case of delays.
2. Never leave medication in your luggage; always carry them with you. (You never know what will come up unexpectantly)
3. Always keep a list of the medications you are taking inside of your wallet or purse.
4. Always keep the pharmacies phone number handy.
5. Always have your doctor's phone number handy.
6. Order a medical alert necklace or bracelet (letting others know you are a transplant patient)
7. Keep regular dosages of medications in organized medicine containers.
8. Keep a list of all allergies to medications or foods.
9. Always keep hands clean when taking medications
10. Always carry bottles of water to take medications.

Most or some anti-rejection medications will be taken for a lifetime. It is extremely important for transplant patients to treat their medications as a part of a normal daily routine. The organ depends on you being responsible for taking your prescribed medications as directed. Get to know your prescribed medications like the back of your hand. You need to not only take your medications regularly; you need to know what each one is for. Once you know the reason for taking the medications, it will change the way you feel about taking them. I am not a person who likes taking medicine. But I realize how important the medication is for my kidney to function. Therefore, I had to not look at taking medicine as a chore. I keep an organizer with me, which helps to make my day run a lot more smoothly. It is always about how we respond to what happens in our lives.

Effects of Anti-Rejection Medications

Patients may experience some or all of the following symptoms with taking anti-rejection medications. I have experienced a few off of the list. Some of the symptoms I experienced with the 1st transplant and not with the 2nd one. My most annoying area has been with the excessive weight gain. The only way I've been able to combat the extra weight gain is through proper diet and exercise. It is important to drink plenty of water, eat fresh fruit and vegetables. Below I've provided a table listing some of the side effects transplant patients may get after taking the anti-rejection medications.

Side effects to Anti-rejection Medications	
• *Weight gain* • *nausea* • *swelling of feet, hands, fingers, stomach and face* • *depression* • *mood swings* • *acne* • *increase appetite* • *Decrease in libido*	• *Insomnia* • *hair loss* • *Extra hair growth in unwanted places* • *anxiety* • *headaches* • *Vomiting* • *Confusion* • *Crying spells*

Below are some habits I discovered helps me keep the weight off:

- I still avoid salty foods. (I am not always successful but I do pretty well).
- I avoid eating sweets (every now and then I still splurge).
- Work out at least three times a week.
- Try to get plenty of rest (learn to take time out for yourself)
- Remain active in pursuing my dreams (happiness is essential to good health).
- Take daily vitamins (ask your doctor what they recommend).

Additional ESRD Resources

National Kidney Foundation
800-622-9010

National Kidney Transplant Assistant Fund
800-642-8399

(UNOS) United Network for Organ Sharing
888-894-6361

(NORD) National Organization of Rare Disorders
800-999-6673

Prograf/Fujisawa Patients Assistant Program
800-477-6472

Prescription Drug Patients Assistance
800-762-4636

American Kidney Fund
800-638-8299

The Transplant Foundation
800-285-5115

Transplant Recipient International Organization
800-874-6386

Rapamune Patient Assistance
877-472-7268

Important Things For ESRD Patients to Remember

- Bring someone with you to appointments (this can help you to remember things)
- Ask for material about all forms of treatments before making your decision (the more informed you are about what is available the better that you are aware in making your selection).
- Monitor and keep track of your blood pressure
- Maintain weight
- Eat proper nutrition (stay away from salty foods)
- Take all medications as prescribed by your doctor
- Never take over the counter medications unless you've consulted your doctor
- Never skip anti rejection medications under any circumstances
- Always keep track of medication dosages written down.
- Make sure that you have clarity on the amount of all medications from your healthcare provider
- Write down any information about your treatments so that you don't forget anything (you will be amazed at how easy it is to forget things)
- Educate yourself about your condition
- Talk to other patients that have experienced what you are going through or another treatment that you're considering
- Become informed about everything involving your health
- Most importantly live life to the fullest!!!

Inspirational Books & Other ESRD Informative Materials

I'm Still Here!	Ted Alan Dyer
Can You Stand To Be Blessed?	Bishop TD Jakes
Have You Felt Like	
Giving Up Lately?	David Wilkerson
Battlefield Of The Mind	Joyce Meyers
Battle Techniques For	
War Weary Saints	Mike Murdock

There are also free videos available through Fujisawa Healthcare to assist you in making a choice about different form of treatments:

Understanding Transplant Issues featuring kidney & Liver Patients *The African American Perspective*

Choices of Experiences Kidney and Liver Transplant Patients Share Their Success Stories

The Basis of Transplant Success

Understanding Transplant Issues featuring kidney & Liver Patients *The Healthy Heart Perspective*

Patients can contact Fujisawa for more information:

Fujisawa Healthcare, Inc
7224 W. 60th St.
Summit, ILL 60501
Or by calling them toll free at 800 477-6472

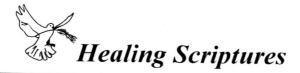

Healing Scriptures

*(Ps 103:3 KJV) Who forgiveth all thine iniquities;
who healeth all thy diseases*

*(Matt 25:36 KJV) Naked and ye visited me: I was in prison and you came
unto me.*

*(Ps 107:20 KJV) He sent his word, and healed them, and delivered them
from their destruction*

*(Is. 53:5 KJV) But he was wounded for our transgressions; he was
bruised for our iniquities: the chastisement of our peace was upon him;
and with his stripes we are healed.*

*(1 Pet. 2:24 KJV) Who him ownself bare our sins in his own body on the
tree, that we, being dead to sins, should live unto righteousness: By
whose stripes ye were healed.*

*(Matt 4:23 KJV) And Jesus went about all Galilee, teaching and
preaching the gospel of the kingdom, and healing all manner of disease
among the people.*

(Psm. 6:2 KJV) Have Mercy on me, O Lord; for I am weak: O
Lord heal me; for my bones are vexed.

Glossary Terms

Acute Renal Failure usually happens quickly and can be temporary. The kidneys can stop working due to such things as loss of blood, a severe burn, infections, medications or certain types of poisoning. Dialysis may not be needed for a short time while the kidneys heal. With acute renal failure, normal kidney function can return after the kidneys heal from the injury.

Cadaveric (Cadaver) Donor Kidney is a kidney that comes from a person who has just died.

Chronic Renal Failure CRF can happen slowly and is usually caused by damage to your kidneys in the form of a disease. Diabetes is a disease of high blood glucose sugar levels. It can cause changes in the structure and function of blood vessels and abnormal metabolism of carbohydrates, fat and protein. Overtime the small vessels of the kidney are affected, causing destruction of the nephrons (the filters of the kidneys).

Dialysis is the process of cleansing waste from the bloodstream artificially.

Edema is swelling caused by too much fluid in the body.

Glossary Terms

End Stage Renal Disease (ESRD) occurs when the kidneys no longer work. In ESRD normal kidney function doesn't return. Therefore, you will need dialysis or a kidney transplant in order to stay alive.

Epogen (EPO Injections) is a medication that assists the body in producing red blood cells. Kidney failure causes the body not to produce erythropoietin the same way it once did when the kidneys functioned normally.

Erythropoietin is a hormone made by the kidneys to help form red blood cells. Lack of the hormone may lead to anemia.

Exchange term used to describe each time a dialysate solution is used in peritoneal dialysis is drained and refilled.

Fistula is a surgical connection of an artery directly into a vein usually placed in the forearm for the purpose administering hemodialysis.

Glomerulonephritis is a swelling of the filters of both kidneys. Sometimes the cause can be due to infection. Involves a slow progressive damage of the kidney function. Early diagnosis is difficult because there are no symptoms in the early stages of this disease.

Glossary Terms

Graft is a surgical connection of an artery and a vein with an artificial tube. The artificial tube will be used for the administration of dialysate solution during hemodialysis.

Hypertension (high blood pressure) damages the blood vessels in the kidneys and reduces the blood supply to the kidneys. If you control it, you may be able to slow down the kidney damage.

Infiltration process by which substances pass into cells or into the spaces around cells.

Kidneys are two bean shaped organs that filter all the waste from the bloodstream.

Live Unrelated Donor Kidney is a kidney that comes from someone who is not related to the recipient.

Nephrology is the study of the kidney

Nephrosis is a disintegration of the kidney without signs of inflammation.

Nephritis is an inflammation of the kidneys

Glossary Terms

Nephritic Syndrome is a non-inflammatory disease. It causes amounts of protein to pass from the blood into the urine. As a result of the loss of protein, large amounts of water stay in your body. This results in overall swelling in your body called edema.

Parathyroid four small round pea shaped areas. Two are located on each side of the neck. The Parathyroid maintains calcium balance in the body.

Phosphorus Binders is medications used to prevent the body from removing too much calcium in the body. Helps to keep the bodies bones healthy and strong.

Polycystic Kidney Disease is an inherited disease. With this disease abnormal sacs, called cysts, develop in the kidneys. These cysts may contain fluid, gas or tissue. As these cysts grow, they block normal kidney function. Cysts may be painful because of the blockages. If you have a polycystic kidney disease you can still urinate in normal amounts, but the harmful waste products aren't removed from the body.

Related Donor Kidney is a kidney that comes from a blood relative of a recipient.

Renal pertaining to the kidney.

Glossary Terms

Transplantation is a surgical procedure of implanting a kidney from a donor into a recipient. Today there are five types of donations: Cadaver, Living Related and Living Non-Related Positive Cossmatch and ABO-Incompatible Living Donor Transplants.

Ureters are tubes that carry urine form the kidneys to the bladder.

Urethra is the tube that carries the urine from the bladder to the outside of the body.

Uremia poisoning of urinary substance in the blood.

Urine is the liquid waste product filtered from the blood by the kidneys.

Glossary Terms Retrieved on March 1, 2004 from *Home Medical Dictionary*

Covering Medical Terms from A to Z (1994) Ottenheimer Publishers, Inc.

AAKP Patient Plan *Phase 1 Diagnosis To Treatment Choice,* Glossary pp.37-40. For more information call AAKP at (800) 749-2257 or email info@aakp.org

Index

Index Concluded

Author's Accomplishments

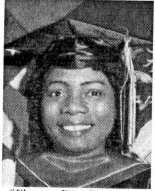

Photograph of Florence Dyer 2002 graduation from the
Graphics Communications Program Baker College-Flint

Dyer is the 3rd born out of nine children. She was born and raised in Chicago, Ill. where she resided until her senior year of high school. She relocated from Chicago to Flint, MI in 1983.

In 1994 while undergoing hemodialysis treatments Dyer became a licensed Medical Assistant. After graduating from the medical program; she worked in the medical field for six years. Due to continuous health problems, she returned back to school to pursue a degree in the *Commercial Art Industry*. In 1995 Dyer married Award Winning Poet, and Author Ted Alan Dyer. In 2002 she received a Bachelors degree in Graphic Communications with a minor in Business Administration from Baker College Flint. Upon graduating, she founded Flo's Productions.

Flo's Productions has professional designs selling across the country. Dyer's designs are inclusive but not limited to the following: designing websites, cartoon animation, designing CD's, murals, brochures, business cards, presentational display boards, magazine layouts, publishing and illustrating books.

In 2004 Dyer received a Masters degree through the University Of Phoenix; from the (MAED) Masters of Art and Education Program.

While attending the Masters Program, Dyer expanded Flo's Productions into a self publishing service and is now publishing and promoting other authors. On May 16, 2005 the (WSPA) Writers & Self Publishers Association was co-founded by Authors David Dicks and Florence Dyer. The WSPA is a program designed to assist aspiring writers into becoming self published authors. In addition to operating Flo's Productions, Dyer is currently hosting the *WSPA Book Review Show.* The review show airs Thursday nights at 9:30 pm on Channel 17 through a local Public Service Television Network. For more information email: writersandselfpublishers@yahoo.com

Words of encouragement from the Author:
There are a lot of things that occur in our lives that are simply beyond any human control, but it is how we choose to deal with these occurrences that determine the ultimate outcome. I learned this from one of my great mentors, who said it best:
It is not where we start, it is where we finish that matters.
---Bishop T.D. Jakes

For organizations that would like Author Florence Dyer to make guest appearances for book signings, speaking engagements, or for more information on publishing books and designs contact:

FLO'S PRODUCTIONS
Call:(810) 334-2837 **FAX:** (810) 785-8419
email: florencedyer@comcast.net
website: http://flosproductions.nstemp.biz

Book orders can also be placed at the following websites:
www.amazon.com
www.barnes&noble.com
www.borders.com

Books Distributed Through Ingram

Appreciation

In 1991 when I started hemodialysis treatments; I did not know what to expect. During that time my younger brother Floyd, had been on dialysis for about four years. He had moved away to Grand Rapids, MI (where he was also attending college). He always seemed to be handling everything just fine. He would come to family reunions and we would talk on the phone occasionally from time to time. But he never really went into details about how the treatments were. Although I was afraid of what to expect he was the only one I knew personally, that seemed to manage quite well. His courage and confidence made my path a lot brighter. I have told him so often, that he has been my biggest inspiration. Floyd let me know all things are possible to them that believe. He has never stopped going on with his life.

Floyd spent twelve years on hemodialysis until receiving a kidney transplant four years ago. He is an accomplished comedian and travels around the world doing comedy shows. I hope that both of our experiences with dialysis and the kidney transplant will inspire ESRD patients to live a very fulfilling life. No matter what you're faced with you can overcome. I know that for a fact, because you are reading this book. We may never get a chance to meet in person. But know in your heart that if you put the Lord first; He has promised never to leave you, nor forsake you. And He didn't stop there, He said that He will be with you even until the end of the age. I never put my confidence in myself or anyone else on earth. There are a lot of people I admire. I have the greatest admiration for my brother. There have been a lot of great mentors in my life. I am even a great admirer of world renowned Pastor Bishop Odis A. Floyd. There is a phrase that he always uses in closing his weekly radio broadcast; He always says, '*Jesus Makes The Difference In Your Life.*' I could not agree with him more. My life is nothing without Jesus in my life. He's the ultimate inspiration for me. I cannot do anything without him. I could not breathe one breath or type one letter. He is my all and all.

Never loose hope no matter what things look like. God is not moved by how we feel or what the circumstances are. He is moved by our Faith. When we believe and act against what we are going through; this moves the hand of God towards us.

Just like in (Luke 8:43-48) *when Luke speaks about the woman with the issue of blood twelve years, she had spent all of her money going from one physicians to another and none of them could help her. But she heard about a man, named Jesus that He would be passing by. She believed if she could only touch the hymn of His garment that she would be made whole.* It was because of her "Faith" that she was healed.

The text clearly lets us know there were others walking beside Jesus that day, the bible refers to a great multitude of people pressed up against Him. To me that says it was not just touching Him, physically that mattered. It says to me that He is touched by what we believe in our heart. That same healing that was available to the woman with the issue of blood back then is still available today for us. He is the same God today and forever, He changes not. I don't care what the doctor's say; just keep on trusting and believing in the Lord. If you don't know the Lord as your personal savior, you can receive Him into your heart right now. Maybe you need healing in your body there is healing available for you now. You can receive the Lord into your heart and healing in your body by saying this prayer out loud with me:

Father, I believe (John 3:16) that *(You) God so loved the world that (You) He gave your only begotten Son, that whosoever believeth in (You) Him should not perish, but have everlasting life.* I believe and I want to regain my health and strength. Forgive me of my sins, removing all obstacles from my life, which would prevent my healing from springing forth. I take authority over sickness and rebuke it and command it to depart right now in the name of Jesus. I believe that I receive the petition that I ask in Jesus name I pray

Amen.

Printed in the United States
40037LVS00007B/208

9 780976 964537